The Ice Cream Diet

PREVENTION'S™

The Ice Cream Diet

THE AMAZING PLAN THAT HELPS YOU:

- **LOSE WEIGHT**
- **LOWER BLOOD PRESSURE**
- **CUT COLON CANCER RISK**
- **REDUCE PMS SYMPTOMS**

Holly McCord, M.A., R.D.
Nutrition Editor, *Prevention* Magazine

St. Martin's Paperbacks

DQ®, Misty®, Peanut Butter® Parfait, Pecan Mudslide®, Royal Treats®, Brownie Earthquake®, DQ® Sandwich, Dilly® Bar, Buster Bar®, Star Kiss®, DQ® Fudge Bar, DQ® Vanilla Orange Bar, DQ Freez'r®, Blizzard®, DQ Treatzza Pizza®, are registered trademarks of American Dairy Queen Corporation.

The nutritional information from TCBY on pages 153 and 248–250 is reprinted by permission of Mrs. Fields Famous Brands.

THE ICE CREAM DIET

Copyright © 2002 by Rodale Inc.
Cover photograph © 2002 by Rodale Inc.

Prevention is a registered trademark of Rodale Inc.

ISBN: 0-312-98548-7

Printed in the United States of America

Cover photograph by Kurt Wilson

Rodale/St. Martin's Paperbacks edition / July 2002

St. Martin's Paperbacks are published by St. Martin's Press, 175 Fifth Avenue, New York, NY 10010.

10 9 8 7 6 5 4 3 2 1

Visit us on the Web at www.prevention.com

NOTICE

CONTENTS

ACKNOWLEDGMENTS

So many people have contributed so much to this book, I could write *another* book just to thank them all! As always, my colleagues at *Prevention* magazine have been incredibly supportive, even volunteering to taste-test more than two dozen ice creams and frozen desserts. (Hey, somebody had to do it!)

I want to especially thank assistant fitness editor Sarah Robertson for all her work on *The Ice Cream Diet*—helping to conceptualize the book, organizing our taste test, collecting ice cream research, reviewing our exercise chapters, and writing about our eating plan for *Prevention*. Editor-in-chief Catherine Cassidy, senior features editor Denise Foley, and assistant nutrition editor Gloria McVeigh somehow managed to clear my schedule so I could devote all my time and energy to this project. And with Catherine's guidance, editorial creative director Susan Godbey, art director Ken Palumbo, and photo director Renee Keith helped shape the book's creative vision.

As always, my fellow nutritionist Janis Jibrin, M.S., R.D., showed pure genius in developing the mix-and-match menus. Anne Egan, Rodale's executive editor for cookbooks, and JoAnn Brader, our test kitchen manager, graciously pitched in to help select and modify recipes to meet Ice Cream Diet guidelines.

Of course, being a "magazine person," I never could have pulled off *The Ice Cream Diet* without the wisdom and guidance of the talented team behind Rodale Women's Health

Books. My heartfelt thanks go to Gale Maleskey, Jennifer Bright, and Pat Dooley, who played an indispensable role in shaping the book's content; to Susan Berg, who is a fabulous and kind editor; to Carol Gilmore, who managed to find just the right-size scoop for the Ice Cream Diet, among other amazing research feats; to Lucille Uhlman and Christine Murray, who provided essential research support; to Karen Neely, who pitched in with the editing at the eleventh hour; to Kathy Dvorsky, who did a masterful job of copyediting all the chapters; and of course, to Dana Bacher, who made *The Ice Cream Diet* blossom from idea into a real book.

I'm grateful, too, to Heather Jackson and her colleagues at St. Martin's Press for pulling out all the stops to produce this book under the pressure of a tremendously tight deadline; to Marsha J. Hudnall, R.D., nutrition director for Green Mountain at Fox Run, for sharing her insight on the issue of "forbidden" foods; and to Brenda Jay Kelly, for serving as an inspiring example that people can eat ice cream *and* lose weight!

INTRODUCTION

"I wish I could eat ice cream every day!"

If only I had a dollar for every time I've heard friends, clients, and family members express their primal cravings for this heavenly food! (My sister Linda, for one, would owe me a small fortune.)

But as anyone who wants to slim down knows, ice cream has tons of calories. Eat ice cream every day, you *gain* weight, not *lose* it. Right?

In fact, that's how the Ice Cream Diet was born. One day during a brainstorming meeting at *Prevention* magazine, several editors jokingly challenged me, the magazine's nutrition editor, to design a diet so they could eat ice cream every day and lose weight, too. None of them thought it could really be done.

But I was intrigued. Could I come up with a real weight-loss plan that included ice cream every day—and more than just a thimbleful? And could I make it healthy, not just a fad diet? It seemed worth a try, especially in light of recent studies using peanut butter, in which dieters appear to have more success when they get to indulge in a favorite "forbidden" food.

In fact, a weight-loss plan featuring a substantial daily dish of ice cream began to make more and more sense to me. After all, we live in a world that bombards us with opportunities to eat delicious, high-calorie treats wherever we go—did you know they even have snack stands down inside

Carlsbad Caverns?!—so diets that ask people to go without these foods seem doomed to fail.

The trick would be creating an eating plan that worked everything out calorie-wise, providing optimum nutrition but building in wiggle room for ice cream every day. After months of calculating, my colleague Janis Jibrin, M.S., R.D., and I have come up with just such a plan. On the Ice Cream Diet, you get to choose a day's worth of meals—breakfast, lunch, and dinner—and an afternoon snack from dozens of menu options that suit just about any appetite and lifestyle. Then you can enjoy a generous serving of ice cream every night and *still* lose weight! As a bonus, the ice cream delivers a nice-size dose of calcium, which pays amazing health dividends, too.

Maybe you're someone who says, "If I take just one spoonful of ice cream, I wind up eating the whole carton." My guess is that you have an eating pattern that's pretty chaotic—skipping breakfast, grabbing something quick at lunch, nibbling a muffin in the afternoon, ordering pizza for dinner, all topped off by a nightly snack-a-thon featuring chips, cookies, and yes, ice cream. If you habitually "starve" all day, it's no wonder you're snacking nonstop at night—and on high-calorie foods that more than make up for any calories you "save" during the day.

But once you start the Ice Cream Diet, you will be eating three healthy, balanced meals every day, plus a mid-afternoon snack. True, thinking about your meals takes a little more effort than going hungry during the day and grabbing snacks at night. But we've kept everything incredibly easy—and the rewards will amaze you.

After just a week or two, I think you'll notice something is changing. The magic of eating three square meals a day seems to be that once you establish this pattern, the bingeing often vanishes. You no longer feel the need to spend the whole night snacking. Registered dietitians have seen this happen over and over in clients who shift to a three-meal-a-day eating plan.

Plus, you'll be indulging in your favorite "forbidden"

food every day—or, more precisely, at night. Knowing you can have ice cream tonight, and the next night, and the night after that . . . well, your urge to finish the whole carton in one sitting should disappear. If for some reason it doesn't, *stop*. The Ice Cream Diet may not be for you. You can still use the menus in this book to lose weight; you just need to choose another snack with the same number of calories as your ice cream treat.

One more thing: Congratulations for deciding to slim down! Losing extra pounds—even a few—will help you feel sexier, more confident, and more energetic. What's more, it will increase your chances of a long, healthy life free of serious illness. But please stop blaming yourself if you weigh too much. It's not your fault.

What made you overweight? For the first time in human history, we have engineered practically all obligatory work out of our lives. Many of us earn our livings sitting. We push buttons to wash clothes. We ride our mowers. Thanks to TV remotes and cordless phones, we hardly have to leave our chairs. The result? Every day, we burn fewer calories.

Also for the first time in human history, we have low-cost, highly palatable food available constantly. In our kitchens. At the mall. At checkout counters *everywhere*. So our natural instinct to eat what tastes good—which kept humans alive when food was scarce—now makes us sitting ducks for all the muffins, cookies, candy bars, and *calories* being thrown our way!

No wonder you've gone into calorie overload, taking in more calories than you burn and getting heavier. No guilt required. Period.

Even though you're not to blame for your weight problem, you are the *only* one who can fix it. You, and you alone, must assume responsibility for eating differently and moving more. That's the *only* way to defeat the environment that is setting you up to gain weight.

Just by picking up this book, you've taken a very important step. As with any weight-loss program, you'll need determination. Lots of it. But you now have in your hands a fabulous blueprint of easy, delicious meals, plus an exercise program, so you can shed those pounds. *And still eat ice cream every day!*

PART I

Lose Weight with Your Favorite Dessert

CHAPTER ONE

Why This Dream Diet Really Works

Sweet and creamy and lusciously satisfying, ice cream is our number-one favorite dessert. We simply can't get enough! As a nation, we spoon up nearly 8 billion pounds of the cool stuff every year. And millions of us wish we could eat it every single day.

The trouble is, ice cream has a reputation for packing on pounds fast. So those who dream of slimmer physiques routinely swear off their double dips in determined pursuit of their weight-loss goals.

But exciting new research just might have dieters everywhere digging out their scoops once again. Why? Because ice cream—when it's part of a healthy, balanced eating plan—appears to help melt away fat, taking off pounds faster than when it's banished to bad-food oblivion. Its fat-fighting capacity seems to have some connection to its calcium content. In one study, dieters who had high intakes of calcium dropped 70 percent more weight than dieters who got less of the mineral. We'll talk more about these amazing new findings in chapter 2.

WHAT'S YOUR PASSION?

When Prevention.com, the *Prevention* magazine Web site, asked visitors "If you could have a daily splurge, which food would you choose?" more than 1,600 people weighed in with their opinions. Of these, a full one-third cast their votes for—what else?—ice cream! The final rankings:

Ice cream	33 percent
Cookies	22 percent
Pizza	22 percent
French fries	13 percent
Cheeseburger	10 percent

WE'VE DONE THE WORK FOR YOU

Make no mistake: If you want to slim down while indulging in butter brickle or fudge ripple on a daily basis, your most critical strategy is to keep a close eye—a very close eye—on calories. That means you must sit down with a calculator and carefully tally all the calories in all your meals and snacks, including ice cream, so you can figure out your exact intake every day.

Hello?! In the real world, who has the time for that kind of planning? Not anyone I know, that's for sure. Indeed, when dietitians consult with clients, the one plea they hear over and over again is this: "Just tell me what to eat!"

So I decided to do just that—to create a plan that specifies exactly what you can eat so you can slim down while enjoying a daily splurge on your favorite frozen dessert. I call it the Ice Cream Diet.

Working with my fellow dietitian, Janis Jibrin, M.S., R.D., I've developed mix-and-match menus—one set for women, the other for men—that allow for a generous portion of ice cream as a bedtime snack. By generous, I mean a whole cup for the ladies, and 1½ cups for the gentlemen. Every single day!

VANILLA RULES!

With all the exotic ice creams now on the market, America's favorite flavors remain surprisingly traditional. Here are the top best-sellers, according to the International Dairy Foods Association:

1. Vanilla
2. Chocolate
3. Vanilla/chocolate
4. Fruit flavors (cherry, orange, peach, raspberry, strawberry)
5. Cookies and cream
6. Nut flavors (almond, butter pecan)
7. Chocolate chip
8. Mint chocolate chip
9. Fudge marble
10. Candy flavors (caramel, toffee)
11. Coffee/mocha
12. Neapolitan

YOUR WHOLE BODY WILL BENEFIT

Now you might be wondering: "If I'm eating ice cream every day, how in the world am I going to lose weight?" That's the beauty of the Ice Cream Diet: Those calories have been factored into the mix-and-match menus! With your ice cream nightcap, you'll be getting a total of 1,500 calories a day if you're a woman, 2,000 if you're a man. That's still 300 to 500 calories below the normal intake—enough for a woman to drop up to 30 pounds, and a man up to 50 pounds, within a year!

Just think: Soon you could look in the mirror and see yourself in that sexy little dress or those really cool jeans that you've been longing to wear. But don't forget how losing weight can make improvements inside your body, improvements that won't be reflected in a mirror but that are vital to your happiness nonetheless. By slimming down on

m Diet—or on any eating plan, for that matter—
urself the gift of a much healthier future.

ce Cream Diet also delivers major health benefits by fulfilling your body's daily requirement for calcium. Based on research over the past 5 years, calcium is shaping up to be the superstar of minerals. We've known that getting more calcium helps protect against osteoporosis and high blood pressure, a key risk factor for heart attack and stroke. Now scientists have uncovered strong evidence suggesting that a healthy calcium intake helps prevent colon cancer and even tames premenstrual symptoms. (We'll talk more about these benefits in part II.)

You may think you get enough calcium from your current diet, but in fact, most Americans run low on this mineral. Only 14 percent of women between ages 20 and 50 achieve their recommended intake of 1,000 milligrams a day; just 4 percent of women age 50 and older meet their goal of 1,200 to 1,500 milligrams a day. (Among women, the average intake is just 652 milligrams a day.) Men should follow the same guidelines for their respective age groups, but in fact, less than one-third of them do.

When you're on the Ice Cream Diet, you won't need to worry about coming up short on calcium. In fact, even your nightly ice cream treat contributes to your daily calcium quota. You'll be getting just the right amount of the mineral—not too little, not too much—every day.

Incidentally, the Ice Cream Diet also provides a fabulous eight servings of fruits and vegetables daily, along with lots of fiber and not too much fat. Your body will love you!

FOUR MILLION WAYS TO PLEASE YOUR PALATE

Following the Ice Cream Diet couldn't be easier. Every day, you select a breakfast, lunch, afternoon snack, and dinner from our practical but delicious mix-and-match menus. Believe it or not, you can create more than four million meal and snack combinations using our menu options!

CELEBRATE!

The U.S. Congress has declared July National Ice Cream Month, with the third Sunday designated as National Ice Cream Day. Beyond these two "official" ice cream holidays, a number of unofficial ones exist as well. Mark your calendar!

National Rocky Road Day	June 2
National Ice Cream Soda Day	June 20
Creative Ice Cream Flavor Day	July 1
National Strawberry Sundae Day	July 7
National Peach Ice Cream Day	July 17
National Vanilla Ice Cream Day	July 23
National Creamsicle Day	August 14
National Spumoni Day	August 21

We've kept all of the options quick and healthy, even recommending frozen entrées and meals at restaurant chains like Wendy's and Olive Garden. You're bound to find foods you love, so you can customize an eating plan to your appetite and lifestyle. No matter what your choices, you'll automatically stay within your calorie budget. So at the end of the day, you can dig into your ice cream guilt-free!

To maintain a reasonable daily intake of calories while enjoying a good-size portion of ice cream, you will need to find a reduced-calorie variety that supplies 125 calories or less in a ½-cup serving. It also should provide about 100 milligrams of calcium, 10 percent of the Daily Value, to help meet your daily requirement for the mineral. Most ice creams have that much calcium per serving, if not more. (If you need help finding a brand that meets these criteria, be sure to check out the comparison chart that begins on page 210.)

Are you convinced that you couldn't love anything but a calorie-rich super-premium ice cream? You might be surprised! Lower-calorie products have improved tremendously from years ago. To guarantee your satisfaction, the *Prevention* magazine staff personally taste-tested a selection of nearly 30 ice creams, frozen yogurts, and ice cream bars.

A BRIEF HISTORY OF ICE CREAM

Long before there were freezers, there was ice cream. The first frozen dessert—a mixture of snow, fruit pulp, and honey—is credited to Emperor Nero of Rome. Making it wasn't easy; snow had to be brought in from distant mountains by slaves. Only royalty ever got a taste of the stuff, and even for them, it was a special treat.

Much of the early history of ice cream is folklore. It's believed that in the 13th century, the Italian explorer Marco Polo learned a method for making ice cream while in China and introduced it to Europe. People began experimenting with recipes for ices, sherbets, and milk ices. Over time, the frozen desserts became fashionable in the Italian and French royal courts.

Once imported to the United States, ice cream earned a new legion of fans that included founding fathers George Washington and Thomas Jefferson. Dolly Madison, wife of the nation's fourth president, even had a brand named after her.

Making ice cream used to be a tedious, time-consuming process that required hand mixing in a bowl. The invention of the ice cream mixer, a wooden bucket freezer with rotary paddles, was a major breakthrough that led to the first wholesale ice cream in 1851. Mechanical refrigeration followed soon after, and in 1926, the first commercially successful continuous process freezer went on the market. Manufacturers could churn out large quantities of ice cream in much less time, making the frozen dessert more widely available and affordable.

The ice cream cone was invented during the 1904 World's Fair in St. Louis. As the story goes, one of the fair's ice cream vendors didn't have enough dishes to keep up with demand. So he teamed up with a waffle vendor, who rolled his product into "cornucopias."

During the stuffy Victorian era, drinking soda water was considered improper, which led some towns to ban Sunday sales of the beverage. That meant no ice cream sodas! An enterprising druggist concocted a legal alternative made from ice cream and syrup but no soda. He dubbed his creation the sundae.

While Eskimo Pies, Creamsicles, Dippin' Dots, and countless other ice cream confections have followed, plain old vanilla remains America's favorite, accounting for about 25 percent of sales. Ice cream makers always assess their competitors' products by tasting the vanilla, because the delicate flavor can't conceal any mistakes.

Even the super-premium devotees found some treats that they couldn't believe were low calorie. (You can see the results of our taste test in chapter 7.)

WHY YOU MUST INDULGE

Perhaps you've gotten this far, and you're thinking to yourself, "I can't possibly try this diet. If I have even a taste of ice cream, I'll end up devouring the entire carton." That might be true—if you continue to deprive yourself. It's a phenomenon that weight-loss experts call the forbidden fruit syndrome.

For many dieters, ice cream is the quintessential forbidden food. "When we tell ourselves we can't have something, we immediately start to focus our attention on it," explains Marsha J. Hudnall, R.D., nutrition director at Green Mountain at Fox Run, a health retreat for women in Ludlow, Vermont. "That increases our desire for it, as well as our chances of losing control when finally we're confronted with it."

When you allow yourself to enjoy ice cream, or any other forbidden food, you actually reduce your risk of a binge, Hudnall says. The key is to maintain sensible portions, and to incorporate the ice cream into a healthy, balanced eating plan—just like the Ice Cream Diet.

PHYSICAL ACTIVITY IS A MUST

When you start the Ice Cream Diet, please, please, please start a regular fitness program, too. Studies show that establishing an exercise habit is essential not just to take pounds off but to keep them off. I don't want you to regain the weight that you lose on this diet because you're inactive. Neither do you.

In part V, you'll find instructions for easy aerobic and strength-training workouts that you can do at home. You'll also get advice on exercising if you're dealing with a specific condition such as high blood pressure, diabetes, or osteoporosis. With your weight and your health on the line, you have every reason to get moving—and no excuse not to!

For now, let's move on to chapter 2, where you'll learn how to figure out your ideal weight—and why slimming down sooner rather than later is so important. You already know that weight loss takes time and effort; changing the habits of a lifetime isn't easy. But if you're crazy about ice cream—and really, who isn't?—then the Ice Cream Diet might be the one that finally works. I'm rooting for you!

CHAPTER TWO

Soft Bellies, Hard Facts

Can we talk? My hunch is that you're reading about the Ice Cream Diet because you're not happy with your current weight and you'd love nothing more than to take off those extra pounds. If you can accomplish that while eating ice cream every day, all the better!

My question for you is, *why* do you want to slim down? If your goal is to feel better about how you look, by all means, go for it! Personal appearance can be a powerful motivator, and motivation is essential to the success of any weight-loss program. But as extra incentive, I want to remind you that slimming down can do so much more than help you slide into a sexy little dress or smart-looking jeans. Simply put, it can save your life.

If you weigh more than you should, you definitely aren't alone. More Americans than ever are toting around too many pounds. Back in 1990, surveys found that 45 percent of adults in the United States were too heavy for their own good. By 2001, that figure had risen to 61 percent. And it keeps getting worse—fast.

Overweight and obesity—defined as exceeding a healthy weight by 30 percent or more—have become a national epidemic, according to the U.S. surgeon general. An alarming 300,000 deaths a year are associated with weight problems.

In fact, the health implications of weighing too much are so serious that in 2002, the Centers for Disease Control and Prevention (CDC) in Atlanta asked the federal government to classify obesity as a disease.

WHY GAMBLE WITH YOUR HEALTH?

What prompted the CDC's request is an ever-growing body of research linking overweight and obesity with a long list of debilitating ailments. If you ever need a little extra incentive to stick with the Ice Cream Diet—or any weight-loss program, for that matter—you might want to contemplate the following long-term health effects of an expanding waistline.

• Adults considered obese are 50 to 100 percent more likely to die before their time than adults who maintain healthy weights. Actually, even an extra 10 to 20 pounds can increase the odds of premature death.

• Being 10 to 20 pounds overweight also raises a woman's risk of heart disease—including heart attack and congestive heart failure—by 25 percent and a man's by 60 percent. The higher a person's weight, the greater the risk.

• Women who gain more than 20 pounds between age 18 and midlife are twice as likely to develop breast cancer after menopause as women in the same age group who don't gain weight.

• People who are between 11 and 18 pounds over their ideal weights have twice the risk of developing type 2 diabetes as those who are not overweight. Carrying an extra 44 pounds or more quadruples the risk. Perhaps not surprisingly, more than 80 percent of people with diabetes have weight problems.

• Adults considered obese are twice as likely to develop high blood pressure as those who maintain healthy weights.

• For every 2 pounds a person gains, her chances of developing arthritis rise by 9 to 13 percent.

Overweight and obesity also have been identified as contributors to respiratory problems like sleep apnea and asthma, as well to depression. And the list goes on.

WHAT YOU WIN BY LOSING

Instead of being frightened by the consequences of weighing too much—a predicament that has ensnared many of us—a healthier reaction is to take control of your situation by starting the Ice Cream Diet today. Happily, dropping even a few pounds can reduce your risk of almost every condition associated with overweight. Consider that a relatively modest 5- to 10-pound loss can help lower blood sugar, blood pressure, and cholesterol.

Of course, the more you lose, the more you gain, healthwise. In a study at the University of Vermont in Burlington, women who dropped an average of 33 pounds lowered their blood levels of a substance called C-reactive protein, which serves as an indicator of inflammation in blood vessel walls. This is a very exciting discovery, as some scientists now believe that fighting arterial inflammation is just as important as fighting high cholesterol in reducing your risk of heart disease.

Want to protect yourself against cancer? Statistics show that between 30 and 40 percent of *all* cancers could be prevented with improvements in eating and exercise habits. Brand-new guidelines from the American Cancer Society, released in 2002, say that maintaining a healthy weight is one of the keys to reducing cancer risk.

If you're a woman with motherhood in your future, slimming down might even increase your chances of having a healthy baby. In 2002, a March of Dimes task force reported that obesity before pregnancy increases the risk of premature deliveries as well as of birth defects such as spina bifida. The task force urges all women who are overweight to get in shape before becoming pregnant.

SURPRISE IN EVERY SCOOP

Okay. You can see why slimming down is your best insurance for a long and vital life. But you're just not sure how eating ice cream can support your efforts. After all, doesn't ice cream pack on pounds?

It doesn't have to, if you follow the Ice Cream Diet. That's because our mix-and-match menus automatically control your calorie intake to keep you in the slim-down zone. And it leaves room for a generous portion of ice cream—1 cup for women, 1½ cups for men—at the end of every day.

What's more, brand-new research indicates that the calcium in ice cream may melt away pounds even *faster*.

Admittedly, the studies so far are very preliminary. But their findings suggest that dieters who get more calcium lose weight at a quicker pace than dieters who get less, even when consuming the same number of calories.

In one of these studies, scientists at the Osteoporosis Research Center of Creighton University in Omaha, Nebraska, tracked 184 healthy women in their early twenties for 4 years. The women who took a 1,000-milligram calcium supplement every day lost significantly more weight than those who were given sugar pills.

These fat-burning effects might be even greater when the calcium comes from foods rather than from supplements, according to researchers at the University of Tennessee. For their clinical trial, they recruited 32 obese adults and asked them to follow one of three reduced-calorie diets. The first group ate no dairy foods but took an 800-milligram calcium supplement every day. The second group got one serving of dairy daily, along with a 400- to 500-milligram calcium supplement. The third group consumed three to four servings of low-fat dairy foods a day, providing 1,200 to 1,300 milligrams of calcium.

The amazing results? After 24 weeks, the group that combined one serving of dairy with a calcium supplement lost 26 percent more weight than the group that only took supplements. But here's the real kicker: The people who got their calcium from three to four servings of dairy foods lost *70 percent* more weight than those who got their calcium from supplements alone!

So how do these scientists explain this intriguing relationship between calcium and weight loss? They can't—not yet, anyway. But Michael B. Zemel, Ph.D., director of the Nutrition Institute at the University of Tennessee in Knoxville, has a theory. When a person doesn't get enough calcium—and most Americans don't—the body releases a hormone called calcitriol. It sends signals to the body's fat cells, instructing them not to break down fat so quickly. "The net result is a bigger, fatter fat cell," Dr. Zemel says. "And bigger, fatter fat cells make for a bigger, fatter person."

Getting enough calcium appears to put a chill on the whole process. And while supplements can do the job, the calcium in dairy foods—like milk and, by extension, even ice cream—appears to work even better. Again, researchers don't know why as yet. But they speculate that dairy foods contain unidentified natural compounds that enhance calcium's fat-fighting abilities.

Think of it as a kind of "food synergy," Dr. Zemel says— much like the dozens of newly discovered compounds in fruits and vegetables that act more powerfully together than separately. "We should be able to accept that in addition to 'classic' nutrients like calcium, other biologically active substances in milk may promote health," Dr. Zemel says.

Though calcium's effects on weight loss need more investigation, researchers are excited by what they've found so far. So are we! Just like the eating plan in the University of Tennessee study, the Ice Cream Diet calls for three or more servings of low-fat dairy foods every day. So you'll be getting at least as much dietary calcium as the study participants—which may help you slim down faster, just like they did. And of course, some of that calcium comes from ice cream—which is fabulous news for ice cream lovers who want to enjoy their favorite frozen treat and lose weight, too!

NO HARM IN NIGHTTIME NOSHING

Does the food you eat after dark—like the ice cream in the Ice Cream Diet—make you fatter? Actually, that's a myth. Research shows that all calories count the same—no matter what time of day they find their way into your body.

The problem is, many people eat little to nothing during the day, then make up for it by stuffing themselves after 5 P.M. If you do that, you are more likely to be overweight—not because of *when* you're eating, but because of *what* and *how much*. After all, when those hunger pangs kick in, it's much easier to tear open a bag of chips and polish off the whole thing than to sauté a helping of broccoli.

By following the Ice Cream Diet, you'll be eating regular meals and snacks throughout the day, so you're not so ravenous at night. And you get to enjoy your ice cream guilt-free, knowing that your calorie intake is under control. The mix-and-match menus take care of that for you!

THE SMARTEST START

Sure, slimming down involves more than eating ice cream, even when it's paired with healthy meals and snacks, as in the Ice Cream Diet. One of the most effective weight-loss strategies also is one of the simplest: beginning each day with breakfast! That comes straight from people who should know—the thousands of successful dieters enrolled in the National Weight Control Registry, founded in 1993 and affiliated with the University of Colorado Health Sciences Center in Denver.

To qualify for the registry, a person must have taken off at least 30 pounds and kept off the weight for at least a year. The actual numbers are even more inspiring. On average, the people in the registry have lost 67 pounds and maintained their weight for 5½ years, according to James O. Hill, Ph.D., a founder of the registry and director of the Clinical Nutrition Research Unit at the University of Colorado Health Sciences Center in Denver. In other words, these folks know how to slim down!

ICE CREAM FLAVOROLOGY

What does your favorite ice cream flavor reveal about your personality? To find out, read through the following "flavorscopes," courtesy of ice cream maker Edy's/Dreyer's. I can't guarantee that they're 100 percent scientific, but they definitely are fun!

Butter Pecan

You are devoted, conscientious, respectful, and fiscally conservative. You hold high standards and show integrity in your actions. You are sensitive to others' feelings but don't wear your heart on your sleeve. You need encouragement from friends and family to share your deepest thoughts.

Romantic compatibility: You are most compatible with those who prefer Mint Chocolate Chip.

Chocolate Chip

You are competitive and accomplished. Although you are competent and ambitious in love and work, you are generous with your time and money, never taking your blessings for granted. You shine in social situations.

Romantic compatibility: You are most compatible with those who prefer Butter Pecan or Double Chocolate Chunk.

Coffee

You are lively, dramatic, and flirtatious—thriving on the passion of the moment. Because you throw yourself into all that you do, you tend to be overcommitted, starting projects without finishing old ones. You thrive on new, exciting ventures.

Romantic compatibility: You are most compatible with those who prefer Strawberry.

Double Chocolate Chunk

You are lively, creative, and dramatic. The life of the party, you charm everyone with your enthusiasm and style. You would rather be with friends than by yourself. You want passion and excitement in your romantic relationships and attention from your mate.

Romantic compatibility: You are most compatible with those who prefer Butter Pecan or Chocolate Chip.

ICE CREAM FLAVOROLOGY (cont'd)

Mint Chocolate Chip

You are ambitious and confident but skeptical about life. You are a realist who prepares for the future; you need a solid plan to feel secure. While your stubbornness is a business asset, it can be a challenge in your relationships. Nonetheless, your loyalty, honesty, and dependability create lasting ties.

Romantic compatibility: You are most compatible with others who prefer Mint Chocolate Chip.

Rocky Road

You are a mix of charm and practicality. You are outgoing and engaging in social situations. In the business world you are aggressive and goal oriented. You enjoy being catered to, and appreciate the finer things in life. You are sensitive to minor slights and respond best to encouragement rather than criticism.

Romantic compatibility: You are most compatible with others who prefer Rocky Road.

Strawberry

You are a thoughtful, logical person who weighs each option before making decisions. You are content and effective working behind the scenes. In relationships, you are often shy and reserved. Once you commit to a relationship, you are loyal and supportive.

Romantic compatibility: You are most compatible with those who prefer Rocky Road, Mint Chocolate Chip, and Vanilla, and with others who prefer Strawberry.

Vanilla

Nothing is plain about Vanilla, nor vanilla lovers. You are a colorful, dramatic risk taker who relies more on intuition than logic. Emotionally expressive and idealistic, you set high goals for yourself and push yourself to meet and exceed them. On the romantic front, you rely on secure romantic relationships that fulfill your emotional needs.

Romantic compatibility: You are most compatible with those who prefer Rocky Road.

Source: Edy's/Dreyer's Ice Cream

And the vast majority seem to agree that breakfast is a marvelous weight-loss aid. According to a recent registry survey, an amazing 2,313 of the registrants, or 78 percent, enjoy a morning meal 7 days a week, while another 287 stop at the breakfast table 5 or 6 days a week. Only 4 percent are breakfast skippers.

"I think a lot of people skip breakfast as a weight-loss strategy," Dr. Hill says. But it's not a good idea. Researchers speculate that eating breakfast helps prevent overwhelming hunger and possible bingeing, later in the day. That's why we've incorporated breakfast into the Ice Cream Diet. With our mix-and-match menus, you'll be able to choose from 30 fast, healthy, satisfying meals every morning. If you haven't been a breakfast eater, our menu options just might persuade you to change your morning routine and take advantage of this proven weight-loss weapon!

WHAT HAVE YOU GOT TO LOSE?

Before we get much farther into the Ice Cream Diet, let's spend a few minutes assessing your current weight so you can come up with a healthy and realistic weight-loss goal. The easiest, most reliable method is to figure out your body mass index (BMI), which takes into account your current height and weight. In the late 1990s, an expert panel of the National Institutes of Health recommended using BMI to measure overweight and obesity. For most people, it's an excellent tool for determining whether they need to drop some pounds, and if so, how many.

If you're into math, you can calculate your BMI manually. Here's what to do.

1. Multiply your weight in pounds by 703. (Be sure to undress before you weigh yourself, and kick off your shoes.)
2. Divide the total by your height in inches.
3. Divide that figure by your height in inches. The result is your BMI.

BODY MASS INDEX						
			HEALTHY			
BMI	19	20	21	22	23	24
HEIGHT (in)			WEIGHT (lb)			
58	91	96	100	105	110	115
59	94	99	104	109	114	119
60	97	102	107	112	118	123
61	100	106	111	116	122	127
62	104	109	115	120	125	131
63	107	113	118	124	130	135
64	110	116	122	128	134	140
65	114	120	126	132	138	144
66	118	124	130	136	142	148
67	121	127	134	140	146	153
68	125	131	138	144	151	158
69	128	135	142	149	155	162
70	132	139	146	153	160	167
71	136	143	150	157	165	172
72	140	147	154	162	169	177
73	144	151	159	166	174	182
74	148	155	163	171	179	186
75	152	160	168	176	184	192
76	156	164	172	180	189	197

As an example, let's say you're 5 feet 7 inches tall (or 67 inches) and 170 pounds. Multiply 170 (your weight) by 703, and you get 119,510. Dividing that number by 67 (your height in inches) equals 1,784. Divide 1,784 by 67, and you get 26.6. So your BMI is 26.6.

The chart above has done the math for you. Simply locate your height (in inches) in the left-hand column, then scan to the right until you find your weight. The number at the top of that column is your BMI.

In adults, a BMI of 18.5 to 24.9 is considered healthy. Overweight is defined as a BMI of 25 to 29.9, and obesity, a

BODY MASS INDEX (cont'd)							
OVERWEIGHT					OBESE		
25	26	27	28	29	30	31	32
WEIGHT (lb)					WEIGHT (lb)		
119	124	129	134	138	143	148	153
124	128	133	138	143	148	153	158
128	133	138	143	148	153	158	163
132	137	143	148	153	158	164	169
136	142	147	153	158	164	169	175
141	146	152	158	163	169	175	180
145	151	157	163	169	174	180	186
150	156	162	168	174	180	186	192
155	161	167	173	179	186	192	198
159	166	172	178	185	191	198	204
164	171	177	184	190	197	203	210
169	176	182	189	196	203	209	216
174	181	188	195	202	209	216	222
179	186	193	200	208	215	222	229
184	191	199	206	213	221	228	235
189	197	204	212	219	227	235	242
194	202	210	218	225	233	241	249
200	208	216	224	232	240	248	256
205	213	221	230	238	246	254	263

SOURCE: National Institutes of Health

BMI of 30 or greater. The higher the number, the greater the health risks.

How do you lower your BMI? By taking off the extra pounds. You can use the chart above to figure out how much you need to lose. Again, locate your height (in inches) in the left-hand column, then scan to the right. The numbers listed under the BMIs of 19 through 24 indicate a healthy weight range for someone of your height. You want to set your goal within this range.

PART II

Amazingly Good Reasons to Eat Ice Cream

CHAPTER THREE
Build Bones That Last

The fact that calcium appears to boost your fat-burning capacity may have already convinced you to try the Ice Cream Diet, with its three servings of low-fat, calcium-rich dairy foods a day—plus a generous portion of ice cream at night! But truth be told, we've only scratched the surface of what this miracle mineral can do for your health.

Of the calcium you consume, 99 percent winds up in your bones and teeth. That leaves just 1 percent for the rest of your body. It may not sound like much, but it's vital to your survival.

Once that little bit of calcium dissolves in your bloodstream, it moves freely in and around the cells of your liver, heart, arteries, and other organs. And it does something absolutely amazing: It enables your nerves to transmit signals and your muscles to contract.

Take a deep breath. The muscles you just used to expand your lungs would stop working without calcium. Your heart muscle would stop beating, too. In short, without that little bit of calcium, your body would shut down fast.

Maintaining the calcium level in your blood and cells is so important that your body uses your bones as a sort of calcium bank, making withdrawals as necessary. The less of the mineral in your diet, the more withdrawals from your bones—which causes them to become thinner and thinner.

Of course, your best bet for slowing the rate of bone loss is to meet your daily requirement for calcium. Unfortunately, few Americans do. Consider that only 14 percent of women under age 50 take in the recommended 1,000 milligrams of calcium a day. Women age 50 and older should be getting up to 1,500 milligrams a day, but only 4 percent do. Women aren't the only ones with calcium deficits: Less than one-third of men satisfy their daily calcium goals.

Even teenagers, who need calcium for normal bone growth, tend to run low on the mineral. Less than one-third of teens get the recommended 1,300 milligrams a day. (The body builds up nearly half its calcium bank during the crucial teen years and continues to form new bone up to about age 25.)

No matter what your age, if you're running low on calcium now, you'll likely experience thinning bones in the long run. And if you have other predisposing factors, you could develop osteoporosis—literally, porous bones that break with very little or no trauma. As many as half of all women over age 50 will suffer a broken bone related to osteoporosis. One way they can minimize their risk is by meeting their bodies' calcium needs.

AN OSTEOPOROSIS PRIMER

Unless you know someone with osteoporosis, you may not realize the misery it causes. It's not a life-threatening illness, like heart disease or cancer. But it can diminish your *quality* of life—especially after age 50, when you're looking forward to being free and independent. Typically, osteoporosis gets diagnosed in women after menopause, and in men after about age 65. But it begins years earlier.

To understand osteoporosis, you need to know a little bit about bone. Normal, healthy bone isn't solid. Rather, it's a series of plates connected by thick, I-beam–like rods called trabeculae. In osteoporosis, these rods become thin, and they

---

HOW MUCH IS TOO MUCH?

On the Ice Cream Diet, you'll be getting calcium in the recommended range of 1,000 to 1,500 milligrams a day. So in case you're thinking of taking extra, perhaps in supplement form, my advice is: *Don't.*

The maximum safe dosage for calcium is 2,500 milligrams a day. Above that amount, this mineral not only can cause constipation and stomach upset, it also can block the absorption of other important nutrients, especially zinc, iron, and manganese. Preliminary research suggests that men with regular calcium intakes significantly higher than the recommended 1,000 to 1,500 milligrams a day may be slightly more vulnerable to prostate cancer.

You really don't need more than 1,500 milligrams anyway. Intakes above that amount don't produce any greater benefits.

---

may be fractured or disconnected. Under a microscope, the diseased bone looks almost like a piece of termite-infected wood, with holes where honeycombs of bone structure should be. You can see why as osteoporosis progresses, fractures can happen all too easily.

Microscopic fractures of the spine—which occur when weakened vertebrae literally crumble under the body's own weight—can lead to chronic pain and nerve degeneration that impairs leg function. It's also responsible for the stooped back that many people still refer to as dowager's hump. In fact, loss of height can be one of the first signs that vertebrae are crumbling.

And any kind of a fall—or even stepping off a curb or sitting down too fast—can fracture a hip, an injury that becomes more difficult to recover from with age. Most people who fracture hips never walk independently again, and many require nursing home care.

While scientists don't know the root cause of osteoporosis, they have identified a number of contributing factors. Family history plays a major role, as does the drop in estrogen that accompanies menopause. The long-term use of steroid drugs for inflammatory diseases such as rheumatoid arthritis can weaken bones, too.

But getting enough calcium can help counteract all of these bone robbers to some degree. And unlike family history and menopause, your calcium intake is entirely within your control.

YOUR BEST BETS FOR BONE HEALTH

Several bone-friendly lifestyle strategies can help reduce your osteoporosis risk. Make these your top priorities.

Meet your calcium quota. You should be getting 1,000

THAT *OTHER* MINERAL FOR STRONG BONES

Although calcium gets most of the attention, phosphorus accounts for more than half the mineral content of your bones. Most people get plenty of phosphorus in their diets, which is one reason you don't hear much about it. But a new study suggests that in some populations, phosphorus intake might be on the low side. At risk are older women who eat very little and rely on supplements for their calcium; strict vegetarians who avoid dairy products and meats; and people who follow very low-calorie diets.

One of the advantages of dairy foods is that they supply both calcium *and* phosphorus. For example, 1 cup of ice cream has 115 milligrams of phosphorus; 1 cup of milk, 234 milligrams; and 1 ounce of Cheddar cheese, 145 milligrams. (You need about 700 milligrams of phosphorus a day.)

If you're relying mainly on supplements for your calcium, be aware that they aren't providing any phosphorus. One recent study found that taking 1,000 to 1,500 milligrams of calcium carbonate daily actually blocked the absorption of about 500 milligrams of dietary phosphorus. That's just one more reason your calcium should come from foods rather than from supplements—and one more reason the Ice Cream Diet is great for your bones!

milligrams of calcium a day if you're under age 50 and 1,200 milligrams a day if you're 50 or older. (Some bone experts recommend up to 1,500 milligrams a day for those 50-plus.) By choosing your meals and snacks from the Ice Cream Diet's mix-and-match menus, you'll be getting about 1,300 milligrams a day if you're a woman, 1,400 milligrams if you're a man. So your body's calcium needs will be covered!

Monitor your D level. Another nutrient critical for strong bones is vitamin D, which stimulates calcium absorption from your gastrointestinal tract. Unlike any other nutrient, vitamin D can be manufactured by your body—in the skin—if you're exposed to the sun's ultraviolet rays.

The question is, are you getting enough sun? Many of us don't, as our lifestyles tend to keep us indoors. In fact, some busy people spend time in the sun only when they walk from their cars to their workplaces in the morning and back at the end of the day.

Experts don't agree on how much sun we need. But those who specialize in skin cancer are adamant about wearing sunscreen during the sun's peak hours between 10 A.M. and 3 P.M. And that, unfortunately, reduces the amount of ultraviolet light absorbed by the skin. No wonder studies consistently show that many Americans have low blood levels of vitamin D.

To complicate matters, very few of the foods we eat on a daily basis contain vitamin D naturally. That's why it's added to milk. An 8-ounce glass of milk supplies 100 international units (IU) of vitamin D—one-quarter of the recommended daily intake, which is 400 IU. (If you're age 70 or older, you require even more D: 600 IU a day. And some bone experts advise everyone 50 and older to aim for as much as 800 IU a day.)

What many people don't realize is that vitamin D is added only to the kind of milk that you drink from a glass. The kind that manufacturers use to make cheese, yogurt, and ice cream is not fortified. So unless you're drinking four 8-ounce glasses of milk every day or getting lots of sun, you may well run low on vitamin D.

solution to the D dilemma is to take a multivitamin/mineral supplement every day. As part of the Ice Cream Diet, we recommend a multi that supplies 100 percent of the Daily Values for most essential nutrients. The majority of multivitamins contain 400 IU of vitamin D. With that as insurance, most people's D needs are covered! (If you're age 70 or older, you may want to look for a 200-milligram vitamin D supplement to pair with your multi.)

Move your body. A couch potato lifestyle contributes to bone loss every single day. When bones aren't challenged by weight-bearing activity, they *automatically* start to lose calcium. (That's the reason astronauts' bones thin so much after even a few weeks in zero gravity.)

Any kind of physical activity is better than sitting. But for all-around bone building, the Power Jump is your best choice by far (see page 204). Jumping rope also seems especially beneficial. For the hipbones, in particular, squats can be helpful (for instructions, see page 203).

Note: If you've been diagnosed with osteoporosis, be sure to consult your doctor before beginning any fitness routine. And see page 202 for the best exercises for you.

MEDICINE CAN HELP, TOO

As important as a healthy diet and exercise are, other strategies can help safeguard your bones, too. For example, your doctor may recommend the following (and if he doesn't, you may want to bring them up yourself).

Get a bone density test. One of the worst things about osteoporosis is that it sneaks up so stealthily. You don't know how much damage it has done until a slight strain or fall causes a bone to break or a vertebra to collapse. Unless, that is, you undergo a bone density test—a fast, painless, and completely safe screening that tells you whether your bones are healthy or becoming thin.

I advise all women to get a bone density test at the first signs of menopause. Those at high risk for osteoporosis—because of long-term steroid treatment, unexplained frac-

tures, or estrogen shortfalls—should have a baseline
ing earlier, in their thirties or forties. The best bone density
test available is dual-energy X-ray absorptiometry (DXA) of
the spine and hip.

THE FACTS ABOUT PROTEIN

Perhaps you've heard that protein promotes bone loss. Well, that's just part of the story. If you dig a little deeper, you'll learn that protein actually is important for strong bones. The truth is, bone loss is a risk only if you're getting too much protein and not enough calcium, says Robert Heaney, M.D., a top bone health expert at the Osteoporosis Research Center at Creighton University Medical Center in Omaha, Nebraska. On the Ice Cream Diet, you'll be getting plenty of calcium, and just the right amount of protein!

In terms of bone health, too *little* protein is a more serious problem than too much. In fact, a particular kind of protein called collagen is a major component of bone. It forms a matrix to hold calcium and other minerals.

Because your body can't make its own protein, the only way to maintain its supply is to get enough of the nutrient from your diet. Not surprisingly, some studies show that people age 65 and older who eat more protein are less likely to break a hip.

Need more evidence of protein's bone benefits? "A recent clinical trial found that among people taking calcium supplements, those with the highest protein intakes had the least age-related bone loss over a 4-year period," Dr. Heaney says. "By comparison, those with the lowest protein intakes had the most bone loss."

In this study, most of the protein came from meat. But for the protein *and* calcium your bones need, the best choices might be low-fat and nonfat dairy foods like milk, yogurt, cheese—and of course, ice cream! A good calcium-to-protein ratio—one that provides adequate protection for the skeleton—is at least 20 milligrams of calcium to every gram of protein. The calcium-to-protein ratio in cow's milk? About 36 to 1!

If you experience a fracture for any reason other than a major trauma such as a car accident, you should insist on a bone density test, no matter what your age. For anyone over age 50, a broken bone should be considered a sign of osteoporosis unless further testing rules it out. Unfortunately, the vast majority of women who break bones aren't referred for bone density tests by the doctors who x-ray and set their fractures.

Please be aware that your health insurance may not cover the cost of a bone density test. DXA may cost several hundred dollars. Several newer screening techniques, such as ultrasound and peripheral DXA, are less expensive. But as yet, they're not considered as reliable (though that certainly may change). Even if you do have to pay out of pocket for your bone density test, it may be one of the best investments you can make in your future quality of life.

Consider drug treatment. If a bone density test shows that you have osteopenia (bones that are thinner than normal) or osteoporosis, you may be a candidate for one of the medications approved to slow or stop bone loss. Currently, the list includes hormone replacement therapy (such as Premarin); bisphosphonates such as alendronate (Fosamax) and risedronate (Actonel); the selective estrogen receptor modulator raloxifene (Evista); and nasal spray calcitonin (Miacalcin). By starting drug treatment now, you just might avoid debilitating fractures in the long run.

But even if your doctor prescribes medication, you still need a bone-healthy eating plan like the Ice Cream Diet. It provides the calcium and vitamin D that enable osteoporosis drugs to work. "You rebuild bone with the calcium, not the drug," explains Robert Heaney, M.D., a top bone health expert at the Osteoporosis Research Center at Creighton University Medical Center in Omaha, Nebraska. "So the mineral must be present for the drug to do its job in the first place."

CHAPTER FOUR

Slash Points from Your Blood Pressure

If you've been diagnosed with high blood pressure, you—and your heart—are going to love the Ice Cream Diet. Our eating plan has a lot in common with the DASH diet (short for Dietary Approaches to Stop Hypertension) now recommended by the National Institutes of Health. Only ours calls for a serving of ice cream every day. Why is that important? Because ice cream contains calcium, which—in addition to its other health benefits—acts as a blood pressure buster.

Anyone can develop high blood pressure at any point in life. But risk definitely creeps upward with age. New data from the landmark Framingham Heart Study suggest that nine out of every 10 Americans middle-age and older are likely candidates for elevated blood pressure readings. So almost every one of us needs to be concerned.

Why? Because high blood pressure is a major risk factor for heart disease and heart attack. What's more, it's the number-one risk factor for stroke—which many experts now refer to as a brain attack. High blood pressure also can lead to kidney damage. But the Ice Cream Diet can help keep your numbers in a healthy range.

T THE NUMBERS MEAN

Your blood pressure is the force of blood beating against the walls of your arteries. When you have your blood pressure taken, you're told it's something like 120 over 80. The first number is the systolic pressure, the pressure in your arteries as your heart beats. The second number is the diastolic pressure, the pressure between beats.

If your reading comes in at 140 over 90 or higher, you have high blood pressure, and you should be under a doctor's care. A reading with a systolic number of 130 to 139 and a diastolic number of 85 to 89 is considered borderline high—maybe not high enough for medication, but definitely worth reducing. Anything under 130 over 85 is considered normal. But to be really in the pink, you ought to strive for 120 over 80 or lower, which is optimal.

What's most scary about high blood pressure is that lots of people have it and don't even know it. That's why it often is called the silent killer. Untreated, high blood pressure makes the walls of the arteries stiff and thick over time. And it makes the heart work even harder, pumping against high pressure. As a result, the heart can become enlarged and weak. Even people with borderline high blood pressure are at increased risk for these complications.

The only surefire way to find out if you have high blood pressure is to check your blood pressure reading. Ideally, you should do this every year, especially if you're in the borderline high range (130 to 140 over 85 to 90) or you have two or more risk factors. These include overweight, poor eating habits, lack of exercise, and excessive alcohol consumption.

If you are diagnosed with high blood pressure, start treatment right away. It can save your life. Shockingly, while most women with high blood pressure know they have it, fewer than one in three takes steps to control it.

Perhaps they're reluctant to seek treatment because they don't want to take medication. What they—and you—may not realize is that many people are able to rein in their blood pressure readings not with drugs but with simple lifestyle changes, including dietary improvements. In fact, that's the first item on the list of recommended treatment options for those with high blood pressure in the mild to moderate range, provided they don't have diabetes or heart or kidney disease.

If lifestyle changes don't do the trick, your doctor likely will prescribe a blood pressure medication. But even then, by following a sensible, balanced diet, you may be able to reduce your drug dosage (with your doctor's approval, of course).

DASH TO THE ICE CREAM DIET

If you're expecting any dietary recommendations to include a reduced sodium intake, perhaps you haven't seen the latest research. True, salt restriction used to be the nutritional gold standard for treating high blood pressure. But as we've recently learned, it works only for some people—specifically, the 40 percent of people with high blood pressure who are considered salt sensitive. For them, consuming salt can raise blood pressure, while restricting salt can lower it.

So far, scientists haven't developed a test to diagnose salt sensitivity. But they have zeroed in on a few predisposing factors for the condition, including overweight, advancing age, and African-American descent.

Just as important, we now know that a blood pressure reading doesn't depend on sodium alone. Other minerals— including calcium, magnesium, and potassium—play key roles, working together to regulate the body's fluid levels. This, in turn, influences blood volume, and so blood pressure.

And thanks to research involving thousands of Americans, we've discovered that the best way to maintain a healthy blood pressure reading is with a diet providing a healthy balance of all four fluid-regulating minerals: sodium, calcium, potassium, and magnesium. That's where the Ice Cream Diet should be able to help.

ıst like the DASH diet, the Ice Cream Diet calls for two or three servings of low-fat dairy foods and eight servings of fruits and vegetables every day. By following those guidelines, you'll be getting abundant amounts of all four blood pressure-lowering minerals in just the right proportions.

THE CALCIUM CONNECTION

Scientists have long known that calcium plays a role in blood pressure, and that calcium-poor diets can raise blood pressure in some people, says calcium expert Michael Zemel, Ph.D., director of the Nutrition Institute at the University of Tennessee in Knoxville. "But now we know more about how and why this happens," he says.

Back in chapter 2, I mentioned that a calcium-poor diet can trigger the release of calcitriol, a hormone that inhibits the breakdown of fat cells. Well, calcitriol has another harmful effect: It pushes calcium into the smooth muscle cells lining your artery walls. (Believe it or not, your artery walls have muscles!) These cells are responsible for blood pressure regulation. When they relax, your blood vessels dilate, and blood flows under less pressure. When they contract, your blood vessels narrow, and blood pressure rises. This is exactly what happens when calcium moves into your smooth muscle cells: It causes the cells to contract.

"What we've learned is that a high-calcium diet actually suppresses calcitriol, so less calcium gets into the smooth muscle cells and the blood vessels stay relaxed," Dr. Zemel explains. Calcium channel blockers, one of the primary categories of medications prescribed for blood pressure, do basically the same thing, he adds.

If you're already taking a calcium channel blocker or any other blood pressure medication, and you're successfully controlling your blood pressure with it, you might be able to gradually taper your dosage as you switch to a calcium-rich eating plan. But changing your dosage *must* be done under medical supervision, Dr. Zemel advises. People who

CALCIUM-FORTIFIED FOODS

Today manufacturers fortify dozens of foods with substantial amounts of calcium—100 milligrams or more per serving. For this reason, you should take an inventory of your diet to figure out just how much added calcium you're getting, so you don't go overboard.

For your total calcium intake, you should stay in the 1,000- to 1,500-milligram range, especially if you're a man. No one should exceed 2,500 milligrams on a regular basis. Above that level, you could become constipated. In addition, some studies suggest that excessive calcium intakes may slightly increase prostate cancer risk.

Among the most common calcium-fortified foods:

FOOD	EXAMPLE	CALCIUM (MG)
Breakfast bars	NutriGrain Strawberry Yogurt Bar	200
Breakfast cereals	Whole Grain Total, 3/4 cup serving	1,000
Energy bars	PowerBar	300
Meal replacement drinks	Ultra Slim-Fast Ready-to-Drink Shake, 11-oz can	400
Orange or grapefruit juice	Tropicana Pure Premium Calcium Orange juice, 8-oz serving	350
Soy milk	Westsoy Plus Plain, 8-oz serving	300
Tofu	Nasoya Enriched Tofu	300

On the Ice Cream Diet, you'll be getting all the calcium you need from nonfortified foods. For this reason, I recommend trying to

CALCIUM-FORTIFIED FOODS (cont'd)

limit calcium-fortified products as much as possible. The exceptions would be if you use soy milk in place of dairy milk, or nondairy frozen desserts in place of ice cream. Then you want the calcium-fortified varieties.

abruptly stop taking their medications put themselves at risk for heart attack and stroke. It's serious business.

If your regular doctor seems reluctant to alter your dosage within the framework of a calcium-rich eating plan, you may want to refer him to www.nhlbi.nih.gov, the Web site of the National Heart, Lung, and Blood Institute. This is the division of the National Institutes of Health that studies high blood pressure, along with other aspects of cardiovascular health. The Web site outlines the institute's recommendations for managing blood pressure, including the DASH diet—and other lifestyle changes.

THESE DIETS WORK!

For proof of just how much the right diet can benefit your blood pressure, you need look no further than the studies that tested the DASH diet. When followed by thousands of Americans, the DASH diet lowered moderate high blood pressure and reduced stroke risk. Even more impressive, it produces results in just 2 weeks. No wonder it's now recommended by the National Institutes of Health as the first line of treatment for mild to moderate high blood pressure.

The DASH diet appears most effective for people who have high blood pressure to begin with, shaving an average of six points off their systolic readings. If that doesn't sound like much, consider this: For every point you lower your blood pressure, you experience a 2 percent drop in your heart attack and stroke risk.

Statistically, the DASH diet is twice as beneficial for

African-Americans as for other ethnic groups. This is important because African-Americans are more likely to develop high blood pressure. (Many African-Americans struggle with digesting milk because of lactose intolerance. If this sounds like you, see chapter 14. You may have more options for overcoming this condition than you realize.)

What's more, brand-new research shows that the DASH diet helps lower blood pressure even in healthy adults with normal readings. So the sooner people adopt this eating plan, the better their chances of avoiding the gradual rise in blood pressure that most experience with age.

HOW MUCH CALCIUM DO YOU GET IN A DAY?

Before you begin the Ice Cream Diet, you might want to take a few minutes to estimate your current daily calcium intake. In general, most Americans don't get enough calcium. But if you're exceeding 1,000 to 1,500 milligrams a day on a regular basis, you should cut back by eating fewer calcium-fortified foods or switching to a multivitamin with less calcium.

Of course, once you're on the Ice Cream Diet, you won't need to worry about counting calcium. That's been done for you!

Milk (300 mg × # of 8-oz glasses)	_____mg
Yogurt (275 mg × # of 8-oz containers)	_____mg
Cheese (250 mg × # of oz; 1 oz = about 1 slice)	_____mg
Ice cream (150 mg × # of ½-cup servings)	_____mg
Total from "Calcium-Fortified Foods" (page 37)	_____mg
Add 200 mg, the estimated amount of calcium in the rest of your diet	200 mg
Multivitamin/mineral supplement	_____mg
Any calcium supplements	_____mg
Total	_____mg

IF YOU LIKE DASH, YOU'LL LOVE ICE CREAM

We couldn't be more excited about these findings. Why? Because the DASH diet and the Ice Cream Diet are practically twins! Consider the following:

- The DASH diet calls for two or three servings of low-fat dairy foods every day, for a calcium intake of at least 1,000 milligrams a day. You'll get even more calcium on the Ice Cream Diet from low-fat dairy foods, including ice cream! (The average American gets less than one serving of dairy a day, by the way.)
- The DASH diet recommends four servings of fruits and four servings of vegetables every day. We've built the same number of servings into the Ice Cream Diet. (The average American consumes half as many fruits and veggies, or even less, on a daily basis.)
- The DASH diet features whole grains, fish, and poultry— foods you'll see lots of in the Ice Cream Diet's mix-and-match menus.

If you have high blood pressure, you can optimize the effectiveness of the DASH diet—and the Ice Cream Diet—by limiting your sodium intake, even if you're not salt sensitive. The Ice Cream Diet keeps sodium around 2,400 milligrams a day, the amount recommended by the American Heart Association. That equals a little more than 1 teaspoon of salt.

In the Ice Cream Diet menus, we've used three asterisks (***) to mark any menu options that are higher in sodium. If you have high blood pressure, choose these foods sparingly. (The menus begin on page 78 for women and page 111 for men.)

Be aware, too, that calcium from dairy foods works better than calcium from supplements for lowering blood pressure—though exactly why isn't entirely clear, Dr. Zemel says. One possible reason is that dairy products contain potassium and magnesium, minerals that are just as important as calcium for controlling blood pressure. That's another

CALCIUM HELPERS

Dairy foods are the calcium superstars, delivering an average of 250 to 300 milligrams of the mineral in a single serving. But some nondairy foods supply nifty little calcium hits that count toward your total daily intake. Don't think of these foods as calcium mainstays, though; you probably don't eat any of them on a daily basis, as you may do with milk, yogurt, or cheese.

FOOD	SERVING SIZE	CALCIUM (MG)
White beans	1 cup cooked	161
Soybeans	1 cup cooked	56
Black-eyed peas	1 cup cooked	41
Sardines, canned in water, drained	2 oz	220
Salmon, canned, eaten with bones	1/4 cup	100
Collard greens, frozen	1/2 cup cooked	180
Kale, frozen	1/2 cup cooked	90
Bok choy	1/2 cup cooked	80
Broccoli	1/2 cup cooked	40
Almonds	1 oz (24 almonds)	70
Figs, dried	1/4 cup	50

advantage of doing the Ice Cream Diet instead of taking supplements or relying on calcium-fortified foods alone.

MORE BLOOD PRESSURE BUSTERS

How else can the Ice Cream Diet help shape up your blood pressure reading? Simply by getting rid of extra pounds, one of the major risk factors for high blood pressure. As I've mentioned elsewhere, losing even 10 pounds can have a significant impact—not just on your blood pressure but on your overall health.

THE NONFAT MILK MYTH

I remember a doctor once told me not to drink nonfat milk because most of the calcium was removed along with the fat. By now, most doctors—and I hope anyone who's reading this book—know this is *not* true. When the fat comes out, the calcium stays put.

You also can lower your blood pressure by exercising on a regular basis, getting at least 45 minutes of physical activity 5 or more days a week. It's crucial to reaching your goal weight and staying there. If you don't already have a fitness routine, we've taken the liberty of creating one for you. For details, see part V.

What else can you do to control high blood pressure, or avoid getting it in the first place? If you smoke, stop. And if you enjoy the occasional alcoholic beverage, follow this rule: No more than one drink a day if you're a woman, or two if you're a man. (A drink is defined as 12 ounces of regular beer, 5 ounces of wine, or a cocktail made with 1½ ounces of 80-proof distilled spirits.)

The amazing benefits of the Ice Cream Diet don't end with reducing high blood pressure and protecting against heart attack and stroke. In the next chapter, you'll find out how this eating plan can help fight one of the most common and dreaded of all cancers: colon cancer.

CHAPTER FIVE

Drop Your Risk of Colon Cancer

Can dairy foods like ice cream help ward off colon cancer? More and more impressive evidence says, "Absolutely!" That makes following the Ice Cream Diet an even smarter move. After all, colon cancer is the third leading cause of cancer deaths among both men and women in the United States.

The latest findings from a number of population studies support the theory that people whose diets are rich in calcium have a lower incidence of colon cancer than people whose diets run low on this mineral. Perhaps the most convincing proof comes from two large-scale studies, reported in the March 2002 issue of the *Journal of the National Cancer Institute*. Both have produced evidence to suggest that calcium can cut the risk of some colon cancers by half.

Since the 1980s, scientists at Harvard University have been tracking the diets and health histories of two huge groups of people: 88,000 women in the Nurses' Health Study, and 47,000 men in the Health Professionals Follow-up Study. When researchers homed in on the calcium intakes of the study participants, they found that the people who got between 700 and 800 milligrams of calcium a day were 40 to 50 percent less likely to develop colon cancer than the people who got less. More precisely, calcium seemed to protect against cancer on the left side of the colon, the last segment of the large intestine.

On the Ice Cream Diet, you'll be getting more than 700 to 800 milligrams of calcium every day. And you'll do it by incorporating delicious calcium-rich foods into your meals and snacks—and enjoying a serving of ice cream, also a calcium source, every night!

MORE MILK, BETTER BIOPSIES

Another convincing demonstration of the power of calcium—specifically the calcium from dairy foods—to inhibit colon cancer comes from groundbreaking research led by Peter Holt, M.D., a gastroenterologist and calcium researcher at St. Luke's Roosevelt Hospital Center in New York City. Dr. Holt and his colleagues were the first to investigate whether consuming low-fat dairy products could afford any protection to people at high risk for colon cancer.

For their study, the researchers recruited 70 volunteers—average age 66 to 67—with a history of colon polyps, small growths that are considered precursors to colon cancer because they often turn malignant. The study participants doubled their calcium intakes to about 1,500 milligrams a day by consuming low-fat dairy products like nonfat milk.

"Biopsy samples taken regularly over the course of a year showed that the increase in low-fat dairy products reduced proliferative activity of cells lining the colon and restored markers of normal cellular differentiation," Dr. Holt says. In layperson's terms, the cells in the colon appeared less likely to turn into something mean and ugly, like cancer. "It was remarkably positive," Dr. Holt says. "The results were quite encouraging."

Indeed, two other intervention studies—both involving supplements rather than dairy foods—seem to confirm calcium's ability to stop colon cancer from gaining a foothold. For one of the studies, people who had colon polyps took either a placebo or a supplement containing 1,600 milligrams of calcium plus a mix of antioxidants (150 milligrams of vitamin C, 100 micrograms of the mineral selenium, and 15 milligrams of beta-carotene). Researchers tracked the study participants for 3 years. During that time, the calcium did not reduce the growth rate of existing polyps—but it did slow the formation of new ones. Significantly fewer people in the placebo group remained free of new polyps.

WHEN GOOD CELLS GO BAD

How does calcium protect against colon cancer? Scientists offer several theories.

"Numerous studies have proven that calcium precipitates—or binds with—bile salts, which are secreted by the liver to help digest fat," Dr. Holt says. Calcium also precipitates free fatty acids, which are created during the digestion of fat. By binding with these compounds, calcium actually turns them into insoluble substances that are . . . well, pooped out of you! This is important, since excess amounts of bile salts and fatty acids irritate the lining of your colon. "They cause inflammation and stimulate cell proliferation, raising the potential for cancer," Dr. Holt explains.

Calcium also influences "signaling pathways" that tell a cell how to behave and how to act toward its neighbors. "Calcium can induce what's called terminal differentiation," Dr. Holt notes. "It can push a cell to mature to its final form, a form in which it's less likely to change into something else, like cancer." The accelerated cell development has major implications for the intestinal lining, which completely regenerates itself every couple of days, opening the door to literally billions of opportunities for harmful cell mutations.

Among its other potential protective effects, calcium helps regulate a process called apoptosis, or programmed cell death. This is crucial to cancer prevention, since cancer cells usually don't die—at least not like other, healthy cells. Somehow they achieve immortality at your expense.

According to a Dutch study, calcium may even reduce colon cancer risk by binding with heme iron, a protein-iron complex that comes from red meat. Heme iron is believed to

MORE WAYS TO BEAT COLON CANCER

Following a calcium-rich eating plan like the Ice Cream Diet is one promising strategy for reducing your colon cancer risk. These steps can help, too.

• Get regular screenings. According to the American Cancer Society, 90 percent of all cancers of the colon and rectum can be avoided, and regular screenings are one of the most effective preventive measures. *Prevention* magazine recommends a colonoscopy every 10 years starting at age 50, or sooner for people with family histories. If you have no known risk factors, you could opt for a flexible sigmoidoscopy every 3 to 5 years starting at age 50. Both tests should be supplemented by a fecal occult blood test every year.

• Slim down if you need to. A person who is obese has a 50 percent greater chance of developing colon cancer than a person who maintains a healthy weight. Obesity raises the levels of hormones that promote the rapid division of cells, which opens the door to cancerous mutations. But the Ice Cream Diet will help take off those extra pounds!

• Eat at least five servings of fruits and vegetables every day. This can lower colon cancer risk by as much as 30 percent. On the Ice Cream Diet, you'll be getting at least eight servings of fruits and veggies every day. The more the better!

• Schedule at least 45 minutes of physical activity most days. Exercise speeds food through your digestive tract, so potential cancer-causing substances don't have a chance to come into contact with colon cells. People who get less than 3 hours of physical activity a week are 70 percent more likely to get colon cancer than people who work out every day. Regular exercise plays a vital role in the Ice Cream Diet. We've even come up with some moves you can do while waiting for your ice cream to soften to a scoopable consistency.

• Find a multivitamin/mineral supplement that contains 400 micrograms of folate, a B vitamin. Most multis currently on the market provide that much, but check labels to be sure. (It could be listed as folic acid.) By taking a multivitamin with folate every day—which you'll do on the Ice Cream Diet—you can reduce your colon cancer risk by 30 percent.

• If you smoke, quit. Smoking inactivates proteins that normally control cell growth. Smokers are 50 percent more likely than nonsmokers to develop colon cancer.

• Cut back on red meat. Compared with people who eat red meat only on occasion, those who eat it almost every day have a 50 percent greater chance of getting colon cancer.

• If you indulge in alcohol, limit yourself to one drink a day. More than that, and you raise your colon cancer risk by 40 percent, compared with someone who imbibes less. Incidentally, a drink is defined as 12 ounces of regular beer, 5 ounces of wine, or a cocktail made with 1½ ounces of 80-proof distilled spirits.

be toxic to the cells of the intestinal lining. But calcium can alter its chemical structure, rendering it less harmful. "One of the biggest risk factors for colon cancer appears to be the consumption of red meat," Dr. Holt observes. "Calcium may help counteract its effects."

Of course, calcium isn't the only substance in dairy foods with possible cancer-fighting properties. For instance, the vitamin D that is added to milk during processing can trigger protective differentiation and apoptosis in colon cells. "But vitamin D seems to work better when calcium is present," Dr. Holt says.

Other components of milk, such as mucins, butyric acid, and conjugated linoleic acid, are attracting scientific attention for their prospective roles in colon cancer prevention. "We don't know all that much about how they work, but we do think they have a possible synergistic effect," Dr. Holt says. "This may mean that dairy foods are better than calcium supplements for fighting colon cancer."

On the Ice Cream Diet, you won't be taking calcium supplements. You'll be getting all the calcium your body needs from foods—including ice cream!

LOVE THAT LOW FAT!

When you get to the mix-and-match menus in chapters 9 and 10, you'll notice that they use only nonfat milk and yogurt and reduced-fat cheese. The reason: Studies of both humans and animals make a strong case for choosing lower-fat dairy products over their full-fat brethren to protect against colon cancer. In one trial, people who drank 2 percent milk had a significantly lower cancer risk than those who drank whole milk. People who drank nonfat milk also showed a reduced risk.

Don't worry, though: Sticking with lower-fat products won't cut into your calcium intake. When the fat is removed, the calcium stays behind. That's good news not just for a healthy colon but also for strong bones and heart-smart blood pressure. And guess what? Calcium may take the edge off premenstrual symptoms, too! To learn more, read on.

CHAPTER SIX

Take Control of PMS

Cravings for ice cream can sneak up on you at any moment. But if you're a woman, you may have noticed that they're particularly persistent at a certain time of the month, right before your period. As it turns out, a certain nutrient in ice cream actually may help alleviate your premenstrual symptoms. So the next time someone raises an eyebrow as you dig into your Rocky Road, you can say that you need it for medicinal purposes—and be absolutely correct.

More precisely, you need the *calcium* in ice cream, which has been shown to tame PMS in three separate studies. The most impressive of these was a 1998 trial led by Susan Thys-Jacobs, M.D., clinical director of the Metabolic Bone Center at St. Luke's–Roosevelt Hospital Center in New York City. It involved more than 450 women between ages 18 and 45, recruited from 12 outpatient centers around the country. All the women had reported moderate to severe recurring PMS.

At the outset of the study, the women were rated for 17 core premenstrual symptoms, including mood swings, depression/sadness, tension/irritability, crying spells, breast tenderness, abdominal bloating, cramping, lower back pain, and cravings for sweet and salty foods. Then they were randomly assigned to take either a 1,200-milligram calcium supplement or a placebo every day for three menstrual cycles. (When you follow the Ice Cream Diet, you'll automatically get at least 1,300 milligrams of calcium a day.)

By the third menstrual cycle, the women taking the supplements experienced a 48 percent reduction in their overall symptoms. Calcium provided relief in all four major categories of premenstrual complaints: emotional upset, water retention, food cravings, and pain. It was particularly effective against depression, mood swings, irritability, and headache. That's good news for women who suffer from PMS—and for those who live with them! And it's even more reason to try the Ice Cream Diet.

CALCIUM, TAKE ME AWAY!

Exactly how calcium relieves PMS isn't fully understood. It may reduce fluid retention and cramping in much the same way it lowers blood pressure, by counteracting salt's fluid-retaining properties and by relaxing muscles. These mechanisms may explain how calcium supplements help ease menstrual headaches, too.

So what's the connection between getting more calcium and easing emotional upset? Most people don't realize that running low on the mineral—which more than a few women do—has long been associated with many mood-related disturbances, including depression and anxiety. But only recently has a shortfall been linked with PMS, as reported by Dr. Thys-Jacobs in the April 2000 issue of the *Journal of the American College of Nutrition*.

From what scientists know so far, calcium appears to influence premenstrual mood through its link to parathyroid hormone, which is produced by the tiny parathyroid glands located on either side of your neck. In general, when calcium runs low, the parathyroid glands release more of their hormone. But levels of the hormone appear to rise even higher just before menstruation in women who are calcium deficient.

According to Dr. Thys-Jacobs, too much parathyroid hormone can trigger behavioral symptoms such as mild personality changes, confusion, anxiety, and depression—quite similar to the emotional woes associated with PMS. So getting your daily requirement of calcium may boost your mood in part by regulating parathyroid hormone.

Perhaps you don't care about the science or theories. If you have PMS, you just want relief! Although that may mean getting more calcium, I'm not suggesting that you binge on ice cream to do it. You'll only be harming your health in the long run.

Instead, let the Ice Cream Diet show how to increase your calcium intake by eating calcium-rich foods throughout the day and indulging in a satisfying but sensibly portioned ice cream treat every night. After about three menstrual cycles, you should notice whether the diet is having any effect on your premenstrual symptoms. In the meantime, all that calcium is helping to strengthen your bones, rein in your blood pressure, reduce your risk of colon cancer—and possibly speed the disappearance of those unwanted pounds.

GOOD FATS TO THE RESCUE

Like calcium, omega-3 fatty acids appear to soothe painful menstrual cramps. These good fats are found in abundance

---

THE FLAXSEED ALTERNATIVE

If you want to diversify your omega-3 sources, you can always try flaxseed, which contains a less potent plant form of omega-3 called alpha-linolenic acid. Take 1 tablespoon of ground flaxseed every day, sprinkled on cereal or salads or mixed into smoothies. Do make sure it's ground; it has to be in order to release its omega-3s. You can buy preground flaxseed in your local health food store, or you can grind whole seed with a coffee grinder.

Store ground flaxseed in the refrigerator. Fresh flaxseed has a pleasant, nutty aroma and flavor, but older seed smells fishy.

in fatty fish like salmon, mackerel, sardines, and herring. But I'm going to show you how you can get your omega-3s from ice cream!

Scientists believe that our modern diet delivers much lower levels of omega-3 fatty acids than our bodies evolved to function on. One of the consequences of this shortfall may be menstrual cramping. Without enough omega-3s, your body produces more prostaglandins, hormones that trigger uterine inflammation and contractions. Research has shown that taking omega-3 supplements can help reduce the severity of menstrual cramps.

To increase your intake of omega-3 fatty acids, you could eat a serving of fatty fish at least twice a week. If you're not fond of fish, you could take your fish oil in capsule form. Look for a supplement that delivers up to 1,000 milligrams (1 gram) total of the fish oils EPA and DHA per day.

Another option—and my personal favorite—is to turn the daily ice cream treat that's featured in the Ice Cream Diet into an omega-3 bonanza! You can do this with a fish oil supplement called Coromega. The consistency of pudding, Coromega comes in two flavors—cherry and orange—in single-dose squeeze packets, just like some condiments. Each packet contains a 1-teaspoon serving with 20 calories and 580 milligrams of EPA and DHA. But no fishy taste!

On the Ice Cream Diet, women are entitled to a whole cup of ice cream every single day. Why not treat your taste-buds and get your good fats, too? Try mixing a packet of cherry Coromega into vanilla ice cream that has softened a bit. Or combine the orange flavor with chocolate ice cream. Or experiment to create your own combinations. What a delicious way to ease menstrual cramps!

Incidentally, omega-3 fatty acids bestow other impressive health benefits—most notably, reducing heart attack risk. So getting enough of these good fats is important even when you don't have premenstrual symptoms. *Note:* If you're on a blood-thinning medication, be sure to talk with your doctor before you start taking any fish oil supplement.

PART III

Doing the Ice Cream Diet

CHAPTER SEVEN

Choose Your Brand

Now comes the fun part: You get to choose the frozen treats that put the "ice cream" in the Ice Cream Diet. As I said right up front, you want to look for ice creams and frozen yogurts that deliver 125 calories per ½-cup serving. The delicious possibilities will amaze you!

We've designed the women's mix-and-match menus in chapter 9 to provide about 1,500 calories a day, the recommended intake for losing a little more than ½ pound a week, or up to 30 pounds a year. After eating breakfast, lunch, an afternoon snack, and dinner, you'll have accumulated about 1,250 calories. That leaves 250 calories of wiggle room for ice cream every night. By choosing a product that has 125 calories per ½ cup, you can help yourself to 1 whole cup—and still lose weight.

The men's mix-and-match menus in chapter 10 have slightly higher calorie counts—2,000 a day, on average. With that intake, most men can take off almost a pound a week, or up to 50 pounds a year. About 1,625 calories come from your meals and afternoon snack, leaving 375 calories for your ice cream nightcap. That's 1½ cups of an ice cream that contains 125 calories per ½ cup.

PUTTING LOW-CAL TO THE TEST

Okay, let's be honest: Ice creams with 125 calories per ½-cup serving definitely fall at the low-cal end of the scale, especially as frozen treats go. And right now I can almost hear all the ice cream purists out there swearing that "if I can't have my super-premium brand, I'd rather not have ice cream at all!"

My advice is, don't make up your mind until you consider two points. First, low-calorie ice creams have improved enormously since they first came on the market. Many of them are downright luscious. Just ask the *Prevention* magazine staffers who took part in an informal but "blind" taste test of low-cal and premium frozen desserts. My colleagues and I—two dozen of us, to be exact—sampled 24 low-calorie ice creams, frozen yogurts, and ice cream bars, plus three premium products.

I know from conducting many taste tests over the years that taste preferences are as individual as personalities. No matter what the food, some people will like it most, while others will like it least. In other words, you can't please everyone—ever.

That's why I was so fascinated by the fact that in our test of low-calorie frozen desserts, some of the *Prevention* tasters liked every single product! And let me tell you, this was a room full of skeptical people. At the beginning, more than a few were ice cream purists, or thought they were. In the end, only two were holdouts.

Even more fascinating, several low-calorie items scored so high that they surpassed the premium products. Our top 10 favorites appear at right.

Now we're not professional tasters. But like the rest of America, we love ice cream. And we've discovered that some low-calorie products can be just as smooth and satisfying as their higher-calorie cousins.

LIGHT ON CALORIES, HUGE ON TASTE

When my fellow *Prevention* magazine staffers and I sampled 27 frozen treats in an informal taste test, we rated some low-cal products even higher than their premium cousins! Our top 10 favorites appear below.

ICE CREAM/ FROZEN YOGURT	CALORIES (PER ½ CUP)	% DAILY VALUE OF CALCIUM
Breyer's All Natural Light Vanilla Ice Cream	120	10
Healthy Choice Premium Low-Fat Vanilla Ice Cream	100	6
Eskimo Pie Vanilla/Chocolate/ Strawberry Ice Cream	110	15
Healthy Choice Low-Fat No-Sugar-Added Chocolate Fudge Brownie Ice Cream	110	10
Healthy Choice Low-Fat No-Sugar-Added Coffee Almond Fudge Ice Cream	110	10
Tropicana Chocolate Dipped Orange 'n Cream Bar	120	10
Good Humor Fat-Free Fudgsicle Bar	60	10
Healthy Choice Low-Fat Cherry Chocolate Chunk Ice Cream	110	10
Edy's Frozen Yogurt Black Cherry Vanilla Swirl	90	30
Healthy Choice Low-Fat No-Sugar-Added Mint Chocolate Chip Ice Cream	100	10

STICKER SHOCK

The second point to consider before you dismiss low-calorie ice creams is this: Have you ever really paid attention to the calorie contents of premium products? The numbers can give you the willies—as much as 310 per serving of Ben & Jerry's Chunky Monkey, or 360 per serving of Häagen-Dazs Chocolate Peanut Butter.

Remember, those calorie counts are for ½ cup, the official serving size on ice cream labels. And we all know what a hoot *that* is. Personally, I don't know of anyone who eats just ½ cup of ice cream at a time.

So to get an accurate idea of what those premium ice creams are doing to your waistline, you need to take the calorie figures on the product labels and double them—at least. For a woman to stay within her 1,500-calorie limit and eat a cup of Häagen-Dazs Chocolate Peanut Butter every day, she'd have a measly 780 calories left over for meals and snacks. Even regular nonpremium ice creams, which average about 170 calories per serving, don't allow very much room for anything else.

Trust me. To eat ice cream every day and still lose weight, you need a lower-calorie variety, with 125 calories or less per ½ cup. The wonderful thing is, you can find incredible-tasting ice creams that fit the bill, just as *Prevention* staffers did. You may need to shop around a little, but rest assured, the ice cream of your dreams is out there.

Besides checking out our list of low-cal winners on page 57, ask for recommendations from your friends and coworkers. And be sure to read through the comprehensive chart on page 210. You can compare calories, fat, and calcium for dozens of ice creams and other frozen desserts before you head to the supermarket.

You'll notice that our chart includes a handful of regional brands. Please don't overlook the regional and store brands available in your area. Many offer low-cal ice creams that are every bit as good as the big-name national brands. One of my personal favorites is Peach Melba from Weis/King's, a local supermarket chain.

Just in case you feel the irresistible urge to indulge every now and then with a higher-calorie premium ice cream, turn to chapter 11. There you'll find a "splurge formula" that allows you to have your fling and stay within your calorie limit. Just promise me—and yourself—that you'll do this only on occasion, no more than once every 2 weeks. The reason: You'll be getting socked with more artery-clogging saturated fat than experts recommend. But as long as you follow the Ice Cream Diet menus—which are low in saturated fat—most of the time, you can afford a splurge every once in a while.

LOW-FAT CAN LEAD YOU ASTRAY

Avoid making the mistake of assuming that *any* low-fat ice cream is low in calories, too. That ice cream you're eyeing may indeed contain only 3 grams of fat per ½ cup (the U.S. Food and Drug Administration definition of low-fat). But it may also be a calorie disaster.

When we did our own sleuthing, we found a chocolate brownie low-fat frozen yogurt that packed 250 calories into ½ cup, and a cherry- and chocolate-speckled low-fat frozen yogurt that weighed in at 170 calories per ½ cup. But we also came across a low-fat chocolate ice cream with 120 calories in ½ cup.

Why the different calorie counts? When manufacturers remove the fat from foods, they must replace it with something else to enhance the flavor, explains Joan Carter, R.D., a spokeswoman for the American Dietetic Association. Usually that something else is sugar and other simple carbohydrates. As Carter says, "They're not adding carrots."

The question is, how much sugar? If it's a lot, calorie counts climb. But if a manufacturer uses less sugar and more calorie-free fillers (including air!), it produces an ice cream that the calorie-conscious can love!

THE LANGUAGE OF LABELS

When manufacturers lower the fat content of their ice creams, they like to say so on the labels. But their products must meet certain criteria to carry the following terms, as defined by the U.S. Food and Drug Administration. (Remember that less fat doesn't mean low calorie! You still need to read nutrition labels for calories per serving.)

Reduced-fat: These ice creams contain at least 25 percent less fat than "referenced products," which must include other brands, not just the company's own.

Light: These have at least 50 percent less fat, or 33 percent fewer calories, than referenced products.

Low-fat: These supply no more than 3 grams of fat per ½-cup serving.

Nonfat: These have no more than 0.5 gram of fat per serving. They're the best bet to be low-calorie bargains.

CALCIUM CONSIDERATIONS

We've designed the Ice Cream Diet to fulfill your daily requirement for calcium, the superstar mineral that protects against osteoporosis, stroke, colon cancer, and PMS—and may even speed weight loss. Some of that calcium comes from your ice cream nightcap. Women get about 200 milligrams this way; men, about 300 milligrams.

Your task—and it's an important one—is to find a lower-calorie ice cream that contains the right amount of calcium. Usually it's easy. But you do need to be aware of a couple of exceptions that may provide more of this mineral than nutrition experts recommend. With calcium, as with any nutrient, a sensible limit is key.

In general, look for ice creams that provide no more than 10 percent of the Daily Value for calcium—that's 150 milligrams—in a ½-cup serving. That will keep you within the calcium range allotted for your ice cream treat. (Remember, that's 200 milligrams for women, 300 milligrams for men.)

So what are the exceptions I mentioned earlier?

Ice creams that deliver more than 10 percent of the Daily Value for calcium per ½-cup serving. I've seen brands that have twice that much calcium—300 milligrams, or 30 percent of the Daily Value. If you'd be having just a single ½-cup serving, then you'd be fine. But the Ice Cream Diet calls for double and triple that serving size (1 cup for women, 1½ cups for men), which means you'd be getting 600 to 900 milligrams of calcium from ice cream alone. Add that to the abundant calcium that we've built into the mix-and-match menus, and you'd be well above your recommended daily intake.

Experts caution against getting too much calcium on a daily basis. The safe upper limit is 2,500 milligrams a day. Beyond that, you could experience constipation or stomach upset. Men, in particular, need to watch their consumption of calcium-rich foods. Though it's quite preliminary, some research has linked too much calcium to a slightly elevated risk of prostate cancer.

This doesn't mean guys should cut calcium from their diets. They need it to preserve their bones and protect against

---

NUMBERS YOU NEED TO KNOW

When you're sizing up a frozen treat to see whether it fits in the Ice Cream Diet, take note of these three measures on the nutrition label.

Serving size: For ice creams and frozen yogurts, it's ½ cup. For novelty items, it usually is one piece. But check to be sure.

Calories: This refers to the number of calories per serving. For the Ice Cream Diet, you want a product that contains 25 calories or less per serving.

Calcium: The amount of calcium is expressed as a percentage of the Daily Value. You can easily convert the percentage to milligrams by removing the percent sign and adding a zero. For example, 8 percent equals 80 milligrams of calcium per serving; 15 percent, 150 milligrams per serving. (Don't try this conversion with other nutrients; it works only with calcium.)

THE FROZEN YOGURT MYTH

You're not alone if you believe that frozen yogurt is healthier than ice cream. But you may be surprised to learn that today's frozen yogurt is only about 25 percent yogurt. The remaining 75 percent is ice cream.

It wasn't always so, says Philip Keeney, Ph.D., a retired professor of food science at Pennsylvania State University. Dr. Keeney still assists with the school's Ice Cream Short Course, attended every year by ice cream industry professionals from around the world.

Introduced in the 1970s, frozen yogurt was simply that: sweetened, flavored yogurt that had spent time in a freezer. It bombed, Dr. Keeney says, probably because people didn't take to the tart flavor.

When it was reintroduced a few years later, frozen yogurt consisted of about 15 to 25 percent yogurt. The rest was mostly low-fat and nonfat ice cream. The revamped version fared better than the original, Dr. Keeney says. "It tasted like regular ice cream, but it was viewed as healthier," he explains.

Even today, some people prefer frozen yogurt to ice cream—whether because of taste, texture, or its persistent healthy reputation. (Some frozen yogurt does contain live and active bacterial cultures, which may contribute to intestinal health.) Like ice cream, though, frozen yogurt can be high in calories. You're welcome to enjoy it as your frozen treat of the day—but be sure to check product labels for the number of calories per serving!

high blood pressure and colon cancer. Experts simply recommend not overdoing it, at least until they know more about the prostate cancer connection.

Frozen desserts that deliver fewer than 125 calories per serving. The fewer calories a treat has, the more you can eat, right? Well, that depends. You *must* check the calcium content per serving and multiply that by the number of servings you plan to eat. If the total exceeds the recommended calcium range for your ice cream treat—200 to 300 milligrams

SHERBET, ANYONE?

Sherbets are frozen desserts made from water, sugar, flavoring, and only 1 to 2 percent milk fat. That makes them lower in calcium. If you're following the Ice Cream Diet and you love sherbet, try to alternate it with a frozen dessert that's a richer calcium source.

With a few exceptions, ices and sorbets contain water, sugar, and flavoring but no dairy, which means they have no calcium at all. By Ice Cream Diet standards, sherbet is a better choice.

for women, 300 to 450 milligrams for men—simply cut back on the number of servings until the calcium level is where it should be, too.

As an example, consider Good Humor Fat-Free Fudgsicle Bars, which have a modest 60 calories per bar. A woman could eat four bars, and a man six bars, without blowing their respective calorie budgets. But they'd be getting far too much calcium, since just one Fat-Free Fudgsicle Bar has 100 milligrams of the mineral, or 10 percent of the Daily Value. A healthier choice is to have just three bars, for 300 milligrams of calcium—within the recommended ranges for women and men.

Another option: Get fewer calories from your ice cream nightcap and use the unspent calories to enjoy another treat that has little or no calcium. Let's suppose you choose an ice cream that supplies 100 calories in a ½-cup serving. If you're a woman, you could eat two servings, or a full cup, and still have 50 calories left over. You can make up the difference with eight Nabisco Teddy Grahams or about four thin pretzels. Likewise, if you're a man, you could pair three servings (1½ cups) of ice cream with 75 calories of another snack, like 13 Nabisco Teddy Grahams or seven thin pretzels.

Of course, the key to getting proper amounts of calories and calcium is not just finding the right ice cream but dishing out the right serving size. Eat even a little more than you should on a daily basis, and you could end up gaining weight instead of losing it. For now, your objective is to find an ice cream that meets your calorie and calcium requirements. In chapter 8, you'll learn the secret of measuring a perfect ½ cup every time!

CHAPTER EIGHT

Start Scooping

"Ice cream? No, thanks. I'm trying to lose weight."

If dieters ever had a rallying cry, that very well might be it. Invariably, they seem compelled to relinquish their right to indulge in their favorite frozen treat, for fear that all that cool creaminess will slide right to their waistlines.

It's understandable, really. I know how easily a spoonful of ice cream can turn into a bowl, and a bowl can turn into a pint or even a whole half-gallon. No wonder so many people resolve to never let ice cream pass their lips again. That is, until the siren song of their favorite flavors proves so irresistible that they run to the corner mini-mart at 3 A.M., spoon in hand.

What dieters everywhere need to know is this: Eating ice cream on a regular basis may help take off and keep off unwanted pounds. In fact, all "forbidden" foods have their place in an otherwise healthy and balanced eating plan that supports weight loss. Research proves it!

INDULGENCE WITHOUT GUILT

Almost everyone who wants to lose weight creates a mental list of foods they feel they shouldn't eat. The problem is, banishing favorites like ice cream, chocolate, cookies, and

THE ICE CREAM DIET PLEDGE

This is very important, so please do it. Repeat after me: *I will never, ever, ever eat ice cream straight out of the carton. Ever.*

What happens when you do? Well, one spoonful inevitably leads to another. Pretty soon, you've hit bottom—literally. That's not portion control. And it's no way to lose weight!

I suggest a much healthier ice cream routine. Just follow these steps.

1. Ice cream goes in a dish.
2. Container goes back in the freezer.
3. You get out of the kitchen.

anything else that pleases your palate only makes you want them more.

"It's human nature. When we deny ourselves things, we become somewhat obsessed with them," explains Marsha J. Hudnall, R.D., nutrition director at Green Mountain at Fox Run, a health retreat for women in Ludlow, Vermont. "And in the dieter's mind, ice cream is the quintessential forbidden food." It's sweet, creamy, yummy—and utterly irresistible. So when dieters refuse even a taste, they often end up on a binge.

At Green Mountain, guests are encouraged to eat whatever they like—even if it's high in fat, sugar, and calories—to defang the power of forbidden foods. What's crucial is that their indulgences occur within the framework of regular, well-balanced meals. The Ice Cream Diet is structured the exact same way.

Most of Green Mountain's guests are accustomed to skipping meals or eating unbalanced meals, then going overboard. (Sound familiar?) Once they realize they can have their favorite treats, as long as they stick with an otherwise healthy diet, something surprising happens: Their forbidden foods no longer hold such allure. Instead of letting feelings of deprivation drive their dietary decisions, many women are able to home in on what they *really* want. They still eat their ice cream, candy bars, and cookies—but they also develop a better sense of when they'd rather have the apple, Hudnall says.

AN ICE CREAM SUCCESS STORY

Enjoying ice cream in moderation, as part of a healthy, balanced eating plan like the Ice Cream Diet, does help take off unwanted pounds. Brenda Jay Kelly is living proof.

Brenda, a 36-year-old resident of Nanuet, New York, grew up on a steady diet of fried chicken and macaroni and cheese—but seldom fruits or vegetables. As an after-school snack, she often downed a plate of bacon, eggs, and waffles.

And nearly every day, Brenda would visit a local ice cream shop for a double scoop of her favorite premium flavors: strawberry and chocolate. "They had to be together," she recalls. The treat made her feel happy and content.

Eventually, though, Brenda's poor eating habits caught up with her. "My weight started to climb after I graduated from college," she says. "From then on, I just gained and gained."

From time to time, she'd try to slim down, following rigid eating plans that promised quick results. The number on the scale would climb even higher as soon as she'd stop dieting. By age 30, she was 82 pounds heavier than during her college days. She had to buy size 24 dresses to fit her 5-foot 3-inch, 256-pound body.

Still, Brenda didn't get serious about slimming down until 1998, when a series of upsetting personal experiences over the course of 10 days forced her to take stock of her situation. She saw photos from a weekend trip and was mortified by her appearance. Then her pants split and fell to her knees as she walked to her car with a friend. The last straw may have come when Brenda, a nurse and psychotherapist, realized that she had developed high blood pressure.

Soon after, Brenda decided to make the journey to Green Mountain, in search of the secret of lasting weight loss. Expecting to be deprived of her favorite foods, she spent the week before her scheduled stay eating large quantities of everything she could get her hands on, including ice cream. "I thought I should fill up while I had the chance," she says.

But through the program at Green Mountain, Brenda developed a new attitude toward food. She adopted a healthy eating plan that included grains, fruits, and vegetables as well as her favorite "splurges." She also increased her physical activity.

"Getting on that eating plan seemed to make all the difference," Brenda says. "I was in heaven. I wasn't hungry. And I was thrilled to learn that I could eat my favorite foods, that I didn't have to deprive myself."

Once at home, Brenda settled into an eating plan that included one frozen yogurt sandwich a day, in addition to those all-important regular, balanced meals. She found the sandwich—which contained 140 calories and 3 grams of fat—to be as satisfying as those premium scoops she once craved. Even better, she could have one every day.

Over the next 18 months, Brenda lost 101 pounds and six dress sizes. She has maintained her weight at about 155 since July 1999.

And she still eats ice cream nearly every day, though not her frozen yogurt sandwich, which no longer is available. She has switched to vanilla and chocolate frozen yogurt—a couple of scoops swirled with a little nonfat milk until soft, served in a pretty teacup and saucer. And whenever friends tease her for going off her "diet," Brenda replies, "I'm not cheating—I'm eating!"

WHEN TOO MUCH IS NOT ENOUGH

Like Brenda, most people can continue to enjoy ice cream while they slim down. But for a small minority, maybe 5 percent, ice cream can act as a trigger food. In other words, it can fuel the urge to eat more and more, explains Stephen P. Gullo, Ph.D., a clinical psychologist and president of the Institute for Health and Weight Sciences in New York City.

Think about your own dietary patterns, suggests Dr. Gullo, author of *Thin Tastes Better* and an expert in helping clients deal with trigger foods. Have you repeatedly eaten whole pints or even half-gallons of ice cream in one sitting? Do you feel unable to change your behavior, even though you've tried? If so, you may need to think twice about following the Ice Cream Diet.

Having ice cream as a trigger food doesn't mean you have some sort of physical problem, Dr. Gullo notes. You're just one of those people whose appetites are stimulated by ice cream's sweet taste, or its creamy texture, or even its coldness.

If you want to try the Ice Cream Diet, you may be able to override your appetite's response by choosing a flavor other than your favorite, Dr. Gullo suggests. Let's say you're partial to chocolate. Buy a small container of vanilla or strawberry, then follow the diet for a week. Are you able to stick with the recommended serving of ice cream—1 cup for women, 1½ cups for men—without going overboard? If so, you should do fine.

Fortunately, Dr. Gullo says, "Most people can keep ice cream in the house and not have an issue with it." Just be sure to faithfully measure your portions, he adds.

THE SCOOP ON PORTIONS

Dr. Gullo raises an important point: For the Ice Cream Diet to work, you must get the right amount of ice cream—1 cup for women, 1½ cups for men—and no more. Allowing yourself even a few extra spoonfuls every day will add up in the long run. You'll sabotage all your great efforts, and you won't get the expected results.

Fortunately, nailing the serving size every time is easy, if you use the right measuring tools. You have a few options.

Serve tennis balls. Conveniently enough, one tennis ball happens to be almost exactly equal in volume to ½ cup. So you might keep a supply of tennis balls in a small cereal bowl or dessert dish on your kitchen counter for a handy visual aid when you're dishing out your nightly ice cream treat. With one tennis ball representing ½ cup, women

SAVOR EVERY SPOONFUL: TIPS FROM A PROFESSIONAL TASTER

Want to get maximum pleasure from every spoonful of your nightly ice cream treat? We asked John Harrison, professional taster at Edy's Grand Ice Cream in Oakland, California—a man who samples about 60 packages of ice cream *every day*—to share his tips of the trade.

Drink some tea. Harrison prepares his tastebuds to pick up the most flavor by sipping a cup of tea to cleanse his palate.

Temper, temper. Let ice cream sit at room temperature for several minutes to soften or "temper" it before eating. Harrison says this adds depth to the flavor.

Lick away. Of the 9,000 tastebuds that dot your tongue, those that sense sweet are right at the tip. So licking ice cream—whether off a spoon or a cone—delivers the most flavor, Harrison says. (If you try this yourself, you may find—as I did—that the real taste "hit" comes when the ice cream reaches the sides of your tongue, near the back.)

Chill out. For true ice cream pleasure, you need to slow down and separate yourself from the buzz of the day, Harrison advises. Try eating your ice cream in the living room instead of the kitchen, for example. "And really enjoy it," Harrison adds. "Let it be an experience."

would need two to measure their 1-cup servings, while men would need three to size up their 1½-cup servings.

Test your scoop. Ice cream scoops come in many sizes, which means the one in your utensil drawer may or may not be ½ cup. To find out, fill the scoop with water, then pour the water into a glass measuring cup. If you get exactly ½ cup, that's great! You just need to level off your ice cream with a knife or spatula before digging in. (Remember, it's two dips for women, three for men.)

If your scoop holds more or less than ½ cup, you'll need to adjust accordingly. That's when keeping those tennis balls on your kitchen counter can come in handy.

Get a disher. If you'd like to purchase a ½-cup scoop to

WANT PICKLES WITH THAT?

Pickles and ice cream. It's purported to be the quintessential craving of pregnant women everywhere, or at least in the United States.

Surprisingly, perhaps, scientists have yet to find any biological proof for this or any other unusual food preferences during pregnancy, says Roy Pitkin, M.D., an obstetrician/gynecologist in La Quinta, California, and editor emeritus of the medical journal *Obstetrics and Gynecology*.

Biological basis or not, Debra Waterhouse, R.D., author of *Outsmarting the Female Fat Cell—After Pregnancy*, reports that in her experience, ice cream is the number-one food desired by moms-to-be. "I know I craved it!" she says.

Just without the pickles.

make measuring the perfect serving size even easier, visit a kitchen specialty shop or a restaurant supply store and ask for a size 8 disher. This utensil serves up just about ½ cup, says Sandee Spicer of Frank Spicer Company, a restaurant supply store in Norfolk, Virginia.

Like regular scoops, dishers—their name originated in the food service industry, where they're used to dish up food—come in many sizes, Spicer says. They're color coded, too, with the size 8 usually in gray.

In our own search, we found at least two size 8 dishers, each with a thumb depress and sweeping blade for easy serving. Frank Spicer Company sells the Vollrath brand on the company Web site, www.frankspicer.com, where you can locate information to e-mail or phone in an order. Also available online is the size D-8 Ice Cream Disher, made by Johnson-Rose (www.abestkitchen.com).

If you decide to purchase your own disher, be sure to level it off each time you fill it with ice cream. Otherwise, you'll be getting more than ½ cup.

TEN MINUTES TO HEAVEN

No matter how you decide to measure your servings, you can simplify the task by taking your ice cream out of the freezer and letting it soften for up to 10 minutes. You're more likely to get the proper portion this way, because dipping is so much easier.

But while your ice cream sits, you don't have to. Set your kitchen timer and use those minutes to burn some calories or complete a simple chore. Do some gentle stretching. If you have a treadmill, take a quick walk or run. Toss in a load of laundry, pay some bills, or wash the dinner dishes. You might even want to try a special 10-minute kitchen counter exercise routine created for this very situation. (To learn more, see page 204.)

Of course, while ice cream is the star of the Ice Cream Diet, the rest of your meals and snacks are important supporting players. Remember, the key to being able to enjoy ice cream every day is to include it in a balanced eating plan. In chapters 9 and 10, you'll find an incredible selection of nutritious and satisfying choices for breakfast, lunch, and dinner, plus an afternoon snack. By selecting your daily menus from these mix-and-match lists, you'll stay on track for weight-loss success!

CHAPTER NINE

Mix-and-Match
Menus for Women

Now that you know the basics of the Ice Cream Diet, get ready to dig in! You'll enjoy easy and delicious breakfasts, lunches, dinners, and snacks, topped off by a serving of ice cream at the end of every day. *And* you'll lose weight!

In developing the menus that appear here, my colleague Janis Jibrin, M.S., R.D., and I took to heart what readers tell *Prevention* magazine, and what clients tell dietitians: "Don't give me concepts. *Tell me what to eat!*" We've come up with 30 or more options for every meal and snack, so you can mix and match as your tastebuds please. Doing the math, you have more than *four million* menu combinations to choose from! With that kind of variety, you certainly shouldn't get bored.

By choosing one breakfast, one lunch, one snack, and one dinner each day, no matter what the combination, you'll get about 1,250 calories. That leaves room for a delicious, decadent 1-cup serving of ice cream or frozen yogurt—250 calories' worth, as described in chapter 7—as your reward. All you need to do is pick the flavor!

With the ice cream or frozen yogurt, your total calorie count for the day is 1,500. For the average woman, that should produce a weight loss of a little over ½ pound a week, or 30 pounds over the course of a year.

A MULTI MAKES SENSE

Even though the Ice Cream Diet provides a wealth of nutrients, I recommend that everyone take a moderate multivitamin/mineral supplement as a sensible nutrition insurance policy. And I'm in good company. The Harvard Medical School healthy eating guidelines offer the same advice.

What should you look for in a multivitamin? The best ones supply close to 100 percent of the Daily Values (DVs) for most vitamins and minerals. You won't find one that contains 100 percent of the DVs for *all* vitamins and minerals; you wouldn't be able to swallow it! If you're over age 50, make sure your multivitamin has no more than 50 percent of the DV for iron, to guard against iron overload.

Check a multivitamin's calcium content, too. The Ice Cream Diet delivers 1,300 milligrams of calcium a day, on average—and it's from foods (including ice cream), which is best. That amount will satisfy your daily calcium requirement, even if you're over 50. So look for a multi with very little of the mineral; some supply up to 200 milligrams, which you don't need. And you don't need a separate calcium supplement, either!

Remember, though, that to take off and keep off those extra pounds, you've got to exercise. Research is proving that dieters who reach their goal weights and stay there work out at least 5 days a week. That's why we've incorporated physical activity into the Ice Cream Diet. Part V will show you how to get fit at home—without joining a gym!

SIMPLE AND SATISFYING

All of the meals in *The Ice Cream Diet* feature favorite everyday foods like breakfast cereals, sandwiches, and frozen entrées. You'll even find choices for McDonald's, Olive Garden, and many other popular restaurants. You can eat out without blowing your calorie budget!

If you find that some of the home-cooked meals suit your

appetite or lifestyle better than others, feel free to repeat them as often as you like. In fact, from a practical perspective, you'll need to repeat them, so you can use up the ingredients you've purchased. That's absolutely fine. Just remember that for maximum nutrition—and maximum health—the more variety your diet has, the better.

We've designed the women's meals to coordinate perfectly with most of the men's meals (see chapter 10), so you and your partner can follow the Ice Cream Diet together. And please note: If we suggest a fruit or veggie that you don't exactly love, or if you have a different fruit or veggie on hand, go ahead and substitute. The modest calorie differences will balance out. Just steer clear of potatoes and bananas, which are higher in calories than other produce.

One of the many benefits of the Ice Cream Diet is that it encourages you to think about your food choices, and to stick with three meals and one snack a day. Following a structured plan like this will help you avoid "eating amnesia," the absentminded nibbling that can undermine any diet's success. Random bites and tastes, such as helping yourself to the fudge left in the break room by a coworker, add up quickly. Before you know it, you sneak a few hundred uncounted calories, which can translate to unwanted pounds.

QUENCH YOUR THIRST

As you enjoy the Ice Cream Diet, remember to drink at least eight 8-ounce glasses of fluids every day. Other than milk, we haven't specified beverages with most of our menu options. If you find plain water too boring, you can substitute sparkling or mineral water, regular or herbal tea, coffee, or diet soda.

Hydration is important for your overall health, and especially for your energy level. Consider, too, that drinking lots of water and other calorie-free fluids helps some dieters stay filled up, so they eat less.

ESTIMATING PORTIONS

When you need to eyeball serving sizes, use the following as your guide.

• A half-cup looks like a tennis ball, or a little less than a woman's tightly balled fist.

• A tablespoon is half of a Ping-Pong ball, or about three-quarters of a woman's thumb.

• A teaspoon is about as big as the tip of a woman's thumb.

GOOD HEALTH IN EVERY BITE

Besides helping you lose weight, the Ice Cream Diet will provide you with good, solid nutrition. By choosing your meals and snacks from the lists of menu options, you'll be getting 21 percent of your daily calories as total fat and 7 percent as saturated fat, on average. These numbers fall within the ranges recommended by the National Institutes of Health to maintain a healthy cholesterol profile and minimize your risk of heart disease. Be aware that the menu items marked with two asterisks (**) are higher in saturated fat. Avoid choosing these meals and snacks only, as you'll exceed the 7 percent cap that's built into the diet.

You'll also be getting at least eight servings of fruits and vegetables every day. That's important, as scientists continue to identify natural compounds in fruits and veggies that seem to have the power to ward off illnesses such as heart disease, cancer, and cataracts.

Perhaps you've heard that you should be striving for five servings a day, not eight. The latest research suggests that more definitely is better. For example, the landmark DASH (Dietary Approaches to Stop Hypertension) study mentioned in chapter 4 found that for some people, 8 to 10 servings of fruits and vegetables a day lowered high blood pressure as much as prescription drugs did.

Incidentally, if you have high blood pressure—or if you're just watching your sodium intake—you should know that our menus supply 2,400 milligrams of sodium a day, on average. This is consistent with the guidelines of the American Heart Association. Be careful not to eat too many of the meals and snacks marked with three asterisks (***), as their sodium content is on the high side. You can lessen the salt in some of these meals by choosing reduced- or low-sodium versions of convenience items like tomato juice, V8, and pasta sauce.

While limiting sodium and fat, the Ice Cream Diet serves up an impressive amount of fiber—25 grams a day, on average. You'll notice that when a menu item calls for bread, it's almost always whole wheat. High-fiber diets appear to reduce the risk of heart attack, stroke, diabetes, and possibly colon cancer.

You'll also notice that the Ice Cream Diet calls for three servings of low-fat dairy foods a day, which collectively supply 1,300 milligrams of calcium, on average. That's good for your bones, your blood pressure, and for premenstrual symptoms (if you have them). It might even speed up weight loss, as you've already learned.

Of course, your nutrient intakes will vary somewhat from day to day, depending on your meal and snack choices. But if you're into numbers, you may want to know that in a typical day on the Ice Cream Diet—including that 1-cup serving of ice cream or frozen yogurt—you'll be getting the following:

- 1,500 calories
- 36 grams of total fat (21 percent of calories)
- 11 grams of saturated fat (7 percent of calories)
- 220 grams of carbohydrates (59 percent of calories)
- 75 grams of protein (20 percent of calories)
- 205 milligrams of cholesterol
- 2,400 milligrams of sodium

GO AHEAD, CHOOSE SOY MILK INSTEAD

You can substitute soy milk in any menu option that calls for nonfat milk. Look for a product that contains no more than 110 calories per cup and supplies at least 30 percent of the Daily Value, or 300 milligrams, of calcium per cup.

- 25 grams of fiber
- 1,300 milligrams of calcium

Just think: You're giving your body the nutrition it needs while treating your tastebuds to the cool, creamy ice cream or frozen yogurt they crave! What could be sweeter?

So pick your favorite foods from the following menus—and then get ready for dessert. Because on the Ice Cream Diet, you can savor a serving of ice cream or frozen yogurt every night without guilt.

BREAKFAST CHOICES

In this list, you're sure to find some foods that suit your morning schedule, not to mention your morning appetite. On average, these breakfasts deliver a modest 330 calories, 5 grams of total fat, 2 grams of saturated fat, 56 grams of carbohydrates, 15 grams of protein, 9 milligrams of cholesterol, 346 milligrams of sodium, 8 grams of fiber, and 380 milligrams of calcium. What a healthy way to start your day!

When choosing one of the breakfasts that feature cereal, you can pour all of the milk into your bowl, or you can save some to drink by the glass or to add to coffee or tea. Similarly, for those breakfasts that don't include cereal, you can have your milk "plain" or mixed into coffee (like a latte) or tea. And if you opt for a breakfast with yogurt, make sure it's a nonfat product that contains about 120 calories per cup, such as Dannon Light 'n Fit.

You can design your own breakfast, if you wish. All you need to do is follow these important nutritional guidelines.

- Aim for about 330 calories.
- Include two servings of fruit (one serving equals ½ cup cut-up fruit or berries, one small piece of fruit, or ¾ cup citrus juice).
- Also include 1 cup of milk, yogurt, or calcium-fortified soy milk, or 1 ounce of reduced-fat cheese.

1. Cinnamon Apple Oatmeal

Cook ⅓ cup dry oatmeal—quick cooking, old fashioned, or instant—in ⅓ cup nonfat milk, ⅔ cup water according to package directions (usually about 1 to 2 minutes in the microwave oven). Top with (or cook with) a small chopped apple, a dash of cinnamon, and 2 tablespoons raisins. Serve with 1 teaspoon maple syrup or honey, and ⅔ cup nonfat milk.

2. Bagel and Cream Cheese**

Spread half of a 2.5- to 3-ounce bagel (for example, Lender's Refrigerated Honey Wheat Bagels are 2.85 ounces) with 2 tablespoons reduced-fat cream cheese. Serve with 1 cup nonfat milk and 1 cup fresh or frozen (unsweetened and thawed) strawberries.

3. Strawberry Slush

In a blender, combine 1 cup (8 ounces) nonfat strawberry-flavored yogurt (no more than 120 calories); ½ cup strawberries (fresh or frozen, unsweetened); 1½ teaspoons honey; a small, ripe banana; 1 tablespoon ground flaxseed; and several ice cubes (add cubes one at a time). Serve with 3 Reduced Fat Triscuits (or 49 calories' worth of another whole grain cracker).

4. English Muffin and Fruit

Toast a whole wheat or oat bran English muffin and spread one half with 1 teaspoon diet margarine (for example, Smart Beat Super Light or I Can't Believe It's Not Butter Light), the other half with 1 teaspoon jam or jelly. Serve with 1 cup nonfat milk and 1 cup cantaloupe pieces.

5. Bran Flakes with Blueberries***

Use 1 heaping cup flaky bran cereal (with about 145 calories and 8 grams fiber, like Post Bran Flakes) with 1 teaspoon honey, 1 cup fresh or frozen, unsweetened blueberries, and 1 cup nonfat milk. Drink any leftover milk or add to coffee or tea.

6. Waffles and Strawberries***
Prepare 2 toaster waffles, preferably whole grain (check label for no more than 170 calories per 2 waffles, as in Eggo Nutri-Grain). Top with 2 teaspoons maple syrup and 1 cup fresh or frozen (unsweetened and thawed) strawberries, smashed. Serve with ½ cup nonfat milk.

7. On-the-Go Breakfast
Pack 1 can Slim-Fast (11 ounces, any flavor) or other meal replacement drink at about 220 calories per can. Take along a tangerine and 2 tablespoons raisins (for example, a small, ½-ounce packet of Sun-Maid raisins).

8. Apple Yogurt
Top 1 cup (8 ounces) nonfat fruit-flavored yogurt (with no more than 120 calories) with 1 medium chopped apple. Serve with 1 slice whole wheat toast spread with 1 teaspoon diet margarine (such as Smart Beat Super Light or I Can't Believe It's Not Butter Light).

9. Hot Chocolate and Toast
Have 1 mug hot chocolate (1 cup nonfat milk, heated, mixed with 1 tablespoon Hershey's syrup). Serve with a slice of whole wheat toast spread with 2 teaspoons diet margarine (such as Smart Beat Super Light or I Can't Believe It's Not Butter Light). Serve with 1 cup fresh or frozen, unsweetened raspberries or other berries.

10. In-the-Car Breakfast**
Pack 6 Wasa crisp bread slices (or 180 calories and 12 grams fiber's worth of another whole grain cracker), 1 part-skim mozzarella cheese stick (for example, Sargento 24-g String Cheese snack sticks, which come in a six-pack), a 6-ounce can of grapefruit juice, and 2 table-

spoons raisins (for example, a small, ½-ounce packet of Sun-Maid raisins).

11. Bran Muffin and Applesauce
Have a small bran muffin (2½ inches in diameter, a little smaller than a tennis ball) with 1 cup nonfat milk, an orange, and ½ cup unsweetened applesauce (for example, a single-serving, peel-top container of Mott's Natural Style Apple Sauce).

12. Shredded Wheat and Strawberries
Top 1 cup shredded wheat (for example, Post bite-size Shredded Wheat 'N Bran or other cereal containing about 160 calories per cup) with 1 cup fresh or frozen (unsweetened and thawed) sliced strawberries and 1 cup nonfat milk.

13. At-Your-Desk Breakfast
Have 1 cereal bar (no more than 150 calories, such as Kellogg's Nutri-Grain bar), 1 half-pint container nonfat milk, and 1 large apple.

14. Fruit with Toast and Jam
Toast 1 slice whole grain bread, spread with 2 teaspoons diet margarine (such as Smart Beat Super Light or I Can't Believe It's Not Butter Light), and a tablespoon of jam. Serve with 1 cup fresh or frozen, unsweetened raspberries or other berries and 1 cup nonfat milk.

15. Muesli and Apples
Top ½ cup muesli (such as Kellogg's Mueslix or other mueslis at about 150 calories per half-cup) with a small chopped apple and ½ cup nonfat milk. Serve with a tangerine.

16. French Toast and Berries
Dip 1 slice whole wheat bread in ¼ cup Egg Beaters or 1 beaten egg white mixed with 2 tablespoons nonfat milk.

Brown in nonstick skillet sprayed with Pam. Top with 1 teaspoon diet margarine (such as Smart Beat Super Light or I Can't Believe It's Not Butter Light) and ½ tablespoon maple syrup. Serve with 1 cup fresh or frozen, unsweetened raspberries or other berries and 1 cup nonfat milk.

17. English Muffin and Peanut Butter
Toast half of an oat bran or whole wheat English muffin and spread with 1 teaspoon peanut butter and 1 teaspoon jam. Serve with 1 cup nonfat milk, 1 orange, and ½ cup unsweetened applesauce.

18. Raisin Bran and Banana
Top ¾ cup raisin bran (for example, Post, Kellogg's, or any other brand with about 140 calories for ¾ cup) with a small, chopped banana and 1 cup nonfat milk. Drink any leftover milk or add to coffee or tea.

19. Cheese Toast** ***
In toaster oven heat a slice of whole wheat bread topped with 2 slices (2 ounces) reduced-fat cheese until cheese is slightly melted. (Check labels for no more than 5 grams fat per ounce, such as Borden's 2% American cheese singles or Cabot Light Vermont Cheddar 50% Singles). Serve with ½ grapefruit and 3 dried apricots (or 6 halves).

20. Peanut Butter Crackers and Fruit
Spread 1½ teaspoons peanut butter and 1½ teaspoons jam of your choice on 3 Wasa crisp bread slices (or 90 calories' and 6 grams of fiber's worth of any other whole rye cracker). Serve with 1 cup honeydew melon pieces and 1 cup nonfat milk.

21. Bagel, Lox, and Cream Cheese***
Spread half of a 2.5- to 3-ounce bagel (for example, Lender's Refrigerated Honey Wheat Bagels, 2.85 ounces

each) with 4 teaspoons reduced-fat cream cheese and top
with 1 ounce (29 grams) smoked salmon (about 1–2
strips). Serve with 1 cup fresh or frozen (unsweetened
and thawed) strawberries and 1 cup nonfat milk.

22. Cheerios and Blueberries
Top 1 cup Cheerios (or 110 calories' worth of other
whole grain "O"-type cereal) with 1 cup fresh or frozen,
unsweetened blueberries, 1 tablespoon ground flaxseed,
and 1 cup nonfat milk.

23. Toast and Eggs
Scramble 1 egg and 1 egg white (or ½ cup Egg Beaters)
in a nonstick skillet sprayed with Pam. (Optional: Scramble with ¼ cup mushrooms and 1 teaspoon chopped scallion.) Serve with a slice of whole wheat toast spread with
1 teaspoon diet margarine (such as Smart Beat Super
Light or I Can't Believe It's Not Butter Light). Serve with
1 cup fruit salad and 1 cup nonfat milk.

24. Cheese Grits**
Stir 4 tablespoons (1 ounce) shredded, reduced-fat cheese
(such as Kraft 2% Milk Sharp Cheddar or Cabot Light
Vermont Cheddar 50%) and 1 tablespoon ground
flaxseed into ¾ cup hot grits cooked according to package directions. Serve with ½ cup nonfat milk and 1
medium apple.

25. Waffle with Peanut Butter
Toast 1 frozen waffle, preferably whole grain (check label for no more than 170 calories for 2 waffles, such as
Eggo Nutri-Grain). Spread with 1½ teaspoons each
peanut butter and honey. Serve with 1 cup fruit of your
choice and 1 cup nonfat milk.

26. Yogurt with Granola and Bananas
Top 1 cup (8 ounces) of nonfat fruit-flavored yogurt (no
more than 120 calories) with 2 tablespoons low-fat gra-

nola (without raisins), ½ tablespoon ground flaxseed, and 1 small sliced banana.

27. Hot Cereal with Apricots
Microwave ½ cup multigrain hot cereal (for example, Quaker, Mother's, or any other brand that's about 130 calories per half-cup uncooked). Use package directions, but instead of using all water, use half water and half milk; in most cases that means ½ cup water and ½ cup milk to ½ cup dry cereal. Cook with 3 dried apricots (or 6 halves), chopped. It usually take 1–2 minutes to cook. Serve with ½ cup nonfat milk and ½ cup unsweetened applesauce.

28. Cinnamon Toast
Toast 2 slices whole wheat bread. Spread each slice with 1 teaspoon diet margarine, ½ teaspoon sugar, and a sprinkling of cinnamon. Serve with 1 cup nonfat milk and a medium apple.

29. Fiber Power Breakfast
Top ½ cup high-fiber cereal (serving size may vary from ⅓ to ¾ cup; look for cereal with about 10–13 grams of fiber per serving, such as Kellogg's All Bran, General Foods' Fiber One, or Kellogg's Bran Buds) with 2 tablespoons low-fat granola, 2 tablespoons raisins, and a small apple, chopped. Serve with 1 cup nonfat milk.

30. Breakfast at the Diner***
Order a toasted English muffin with 2 servings Egg Beaters prepared in very little margarine (it doesn't hurt to ask). Also, order a cup of fruit salad and a glass of nonfat milk.

LUNCH CHOICES

Whether you eat lunch at work, on the run, or at home, you're bound to find something to your liking here. The average nutrient breakdown for these menu options is as follows: 365 calories, 11 grams of total fat, 4 grams of saturated fat, 45 grams of carbohydrates, 21 grams of protein, 40 milligrams of cholesterol, 889 milligrams of sodium, 7 grams of fiber, 236 milligrams of calcium.

If you'd prefer to create your own lunch, it should meet two important nutritional criteria.

- It should supply about 365 calories.
- It should allow for two servings of vegetables (one serving equals 1 cup of raw leafy greens; ½ cup other vegetables, cooked or raw; or ¾ cup tomato or vegetable juice).

Lunch on the Job

The following choices are lunchtime mainstays for some of the fittest *Prevention* staffers. Many of these meals can be prepared at home and brown-bagged for work. If your workplace has a refrigerator and a microwave, frozen entrées are especially convenient. And their taste has come a *long* way!

1. Tupperware Tuna, Bean, and Corn Salad

In a plastic container with a lid, combine half of a 6-ounce can of drained, water-packed tuna with ⅓ cup rinsed canned beans (garbanzo or cannellini beans are good choices here) and ⅓ cup canned or frozen corn. Add ½ cup halved cherry tomatoes and ½ cup chopped green or red pepper. Toss with 1 tablespoon Italian dressing. (Optional: Add 1–2 tablespoons fresh parsley, basil, or dill.)

2. Chicken Enchilada**

Microwave according to package directions Lean Cuisine Chicken Enchilada Suiza with Mexican-Style Rice, Smart Ones Chicken Enchilada Suiza, or similar frozen meal (check labels for about 260–280 calories, 6–9 grams fat). Serve with 1 cup cucumber slices or other vegetable of your choice and a half-cup of nonfat milk.

3. Ham and Cheese on Rye** ***

Spread 2 slices of rye bread with mustard to taste. Fill sandwich with 2 slices (2 ounces) lean ham sliced for sandwiches (check label for no more than 2 grams of fat per ounce) and 1 slice (1 ounce) reduced-fat cheese (less than 5 grams per slice, such as Borden's 2% American cheese singles or Cabot Light Vermont Cheddar 50% Singles), 3 slices tomato, and 1 slice romaine lettuce. Serve with ½ cup baby carrots.

4. A Taste of Italy**

Microwave according to package directions Lean Cuisine Everyday Favorites Cheese Ravioli or similar frozen meal (check label for 260–280 calories, 6–9 grams fat). Add a cup of raw vegetables of your choice and a half-cup of nonfat milk.

5. Bean Burrito

Microwave according to package directions Amy's Bean and Rice Burrito, Amy's Bean and Cheese Burrito, or similar frozen pocket (check labels for 260–280 calories, 6–9 grams fat). Serve with 1 cup celery sticks or other vegetable of your choice.

6. Roast Beef Sandwich***

Spread 2 slices whole wheat bread with 1 teaspoon reduced-fat mayonnaise each, plus mustard to taste (horseradish mustard tastes even better with this sandwich). Fill with 2 slices (2 ounces) lean roast beef sliced for sandwiches, 4 slices tomato, and a piece of romaine lettuce. Serve with a 6-ounce can of V8.

7. Your Favorite Chicken Lunch

Microwave according to package directions a chicken-based frozen entrée such as Smart Ones Fire-Grilled Chicken and Vegetables or similar frozen meal (check label for 260–280 calories, 6–9 grams fat). Add a cup of raw vegetables of your choice and a half-cup of nonfat milk.

8. Tuna Salad Sandwich***

Combine 1 tablespoon reduced-fat mayonnaise and ½ teaspoon mustard with half of a 6-ounce can of tuna. Make sandwich with 2 slices whole wheat bread, 3 slices tomato, and 2 slices romaine lettuce. Serve with a 6-ounce can of V8.

9. South of the Border

Microwave according to package directions Smart Ones Fajita Chicken Supreme, Amy's Black Bean Enchilada Whole Meal, or similar frozen meal (check label for 260–280 calories, 6–9 grams fat). Add a cup of raw vegetables of your choice and a half-cup nonfat milk.

10. Peanut Butter and Jelly

Spread 1 slice of whole wheat bread with 1½ tablespoons peanut butter and 2 tablespoons jelly or jam. Top with a second slice of whole wheat bread. Serve with 1-cup mix of celery sticks and baby carrots.

11. Ready for Beef

Microwave according to package directions Lean Cuisine Southern Beef Tips or similar frozen meal (check label for 260–280 calories, 6–9 grams fat). Add a cup of raw vegetables of your choice and a half-cup of nonfat milk.

Lunch on the Go

Maybe you're using your lunch hour to run errands. Then again, maybe you just need to get *out*. Either way, you'll find these choices perfect.

12. A Stop at Subway**

Order a 6-inch Subway Veggie Delite on wheat bread with 2 servings (4 triangles) cheese of any type and 1 tablespoon Light Mayo, Honey Mustard, or Southwest Dressing. Make sure they absolutely stuff your sandwich with veggies—ask for extra tomatoes or peppers. Or have the Subway Turkey Breast and Bacon Wrap with a Veggie

Delite salad and use 1 tablespoon Fat-free Italian dressing. Or have the Subway Deli Tuna Sandwich ("deli" sandwiches are on smaller rolls, not subs) with a Veggie Delite salad and use 1 tablespoon Fat-free Italian dressing.

13. Fast Food Burgers**

Order the smallest burger or cheeseburger on the menu—which usually means the "regular" size. Have mustard and ketchup, but no mayonnaise. (Hamburger: Burger King, Wendy's, Hardee's, or McDonald's. Cheeseburger: Wendy's or McDonald's only.) Take with you a sandwich bag of 1 cup baby carrots (or other vegetable).

14. Grilled Chicken Sandwich

Have Wendy's Grilled Chicken Sandwich, the KFC Tender Roast Sandwich without sauce, or the KFC Honey BBQ Sandwich. Ask for just a dab of mayonnaise or use ½ tablespoon at the most. Take with you a sandwich bag of 1 cup red pepper slices (or other vegetable). (Note: Chicken sandwiches at Burger King and McDonald's are too high in calories.)

15. A Stop at Taco Bell**

Order the Taco Bell Chili Cheese Burrito or the Gordita Supreme Chicken. Take with you a sandwich bag of 1 cup celery and carrot sticks, or other vegetable.

16. At the Salad Bar

Take 1 cup mixed greens or romaine lettuce, 3 tablespoons garbanzo beans, and 1½ cups chopped raw (plain, not marinated) vegetables of your choice (tomatoes, shredded carrots, cucumber slices, etc.) tossed with 3 tablespoons reduced-calorie dressing. Choose one of the following: ½ cup (8 tablespoons) cottage cheese, or heaping half-cup tuna (plain, no mayonnaise). Top with either 2 tablespoons chopped egg or 2 tablespoons shredded cheese. Serve with 1 slice whole wheat bread.

17. At the Salad Bar, Vegetarian-Style

Take 1 cup mixed greens or romaine lettuce and ½ cup beans (such as garbanzo beans or pinto beans), ¼ cup plain or marinated tofu (not deep fried), 1½ cups chopped raw (plain, not marinated) vegetables of your choice, 1½ tablespoons regular dressing, or 3 table-spoons reduced-calorie dressing. Serve with 1 slice whole wheat bread.

18. Grilled Chicken Caesar Salad

Many restaurants use about 6 ounces of chicken; you want to eat about 2½ ounces, slightly smaller than a deck of cards. (In most cases that means you'll have chicken to take home in a doggy bag—those chicken slices will come in handy for some of the other lunches and dinners in this plan!) Eat 2 or more cups greens. Ask for dressing on the side; use 1½ tablespoons. Top with 3 tablespoons croutons (2 tablespoons of the really greasy type).

19. A Stop at Arby's** ***

Order the Arby's Junior Roast Beef Sandwich and a Side Salad. Use 2 tablespoons reduced-calorie Italian or reduced-calorie Buttermilk dressing.

Lunch at Home

Having access to a kitchen widens your choices of healthy, satisfying lunches. And these can be ready fast!

20. Veggie Cheeseburger

Microwave a veggie burger according to package direc-tions. Choose patties in the 110–130 calorie range (such as The Original Gardenburger or Amy's California Veg-gie Burger). When nearly cooked, top burger with 1 slice (1 ounce) of reduced-fat cheese (less than 5 grams fat per slice, like Borden's 2% American cheese singles or Cabot Light Vermont Cheddar 50% Singles) and melt. Place on a whole grain bun spread with mustard and ketchup to taste. Add 3 slices tomato and 2 slices romaine lettuce. Serve with ½ cup red pepper strips or other vegetable of your choice.

21. Soup and Half a Sandwich

Heat ¾ cup black bean soup (or 130 calories of other bean soups). Spread 1 slice whole wheat bread, cut in half, with mustard to taste. Pile on 1 slice (1 ounce) turkey breast sliced for sandwiches (check label for no more than 2 grams of fat per ounce) and a half-slice (½ ounce) reduced-fat cheese (less than 5 grams of fat per slice, such as Borden's 2% American cheese singles or Cabot Light Vermont Cheddar 50% Singles). Serve with 1 cup broccoli florets dipped in 2 tablespoons reduced-calorie ranch dressing.

22. Homemade Bean Burrito

Top a warmed 8-inch tortilla (whole wheat is best, such as Cedarlane brand) with ⅓ cup canned pinto or black beans, partly mashed, 4 tablespoons (1 ounce) shredded reduced-fat Cheddar cheese (such as Kraft 2% Milk Sharp Cheddar or Cabot Light Vermont Cheddar 50%) and 3 tablespoons salsa. Roll and serve. Add 1 cup baby carrots.

23. Spinach Bleu Cheese Salad

Toss together 2 cups spinach (save time by buying pre-washed bagged spinach) and 1 small tomato cut in wedges or 6 cherry tomatoes. Top with 2 tablespoons crumbled bleu cheese; 1 hard-boiled egg, sliced; 3 tablespoons garbanzo beans; and 1½ tablespoons fat-free salad dressing of your choice. Serve with 3 Wasa crisp bread slices (or 90 calories and 6 grams fiber's worth of another whole rye cracker).

24. Stuffed Pockets and Soup

Microwave according to package directions Lean Pockets (Turkey, Broccoli, and Cheese or Chicken Broccoli

Supreme) or Amy's (Vegetarian Pizza in a Pocket, Broccoli and Cheese in a Pocket, or Soy Cheese Veggie Pizza in a Pocket. Check label for 250–280 calories, 7–10 grams fat). Serve with ⅔ cup lentil soup (canned is fine) heated with 1 cup fresh spinach (get prewashed, bagged spinach for convenience).

25. Grilled Cheese and Tomato Sandwich**
Between 2 slices whole wheat bread place 2 slices (2 ounces) reduced-fat cheese (check label for no more than 5 grams fat per slice, as in Borden's 2% American cheese singles or Cabot Light Vermont Cheddar 50% Singles) and 3 slices of tomato. Grill on a nonstick frying pan sprayed with Pam or in the toaster oven until melted. Serve with 1 cup raw vegetables of your choice: cherry tomatoes, green or red pepper slices, baby carrots, etc.

26. Black Bean Soup with Sour Cream**
To 1 cup black bean soup (or 170 calories of other bean soups) add 1 cup fresh spinach (save time by buying it prewashed and bagged). Heat until spinach wilts down. Top with 2 tablespoons reduced-fat sour cream. Serve with ½ cup baby carrots, 4 Reduced Fat Triscuits (or 65 calories' worth of another whole grain cracker), and ½ ounce reduced-fat Cheddar cheese (such as Kraft 2% Milk Sharp Cheddar or Cabot Light Vermont Cheddar 50%).

27. Pita Vegetable Pizza**
Slice a 6½-inch whole wheat pita (about 170 calories) lengthwise to produce 2 rounds. Spread each round with 1½ tablespoons pizza sauce or thick spaghetti sauce; ¼ cup chopped mushrooms, zucchini, peppers or other vegetables; and 4 tablespoons (1 ounce) shredded part-skim mozzarella. Heat in oven or toaster oven at 350°F for 8 minutes or until mozzarella just melts. Serve with ½ cup celery sticks.

28. Baked Potato, Broccoli, and Cheese
Top 1 baked potato (2⅓ inches in diameter and 4¾ inches long) with 4 tablespoons (1 ounce) shredded reduced-fat Cheddar cheese (such as Kraft 2% Milk Sharp Cheddar or Cabot Light Vermont Cheddar 50%) and 1 cup cooked chopped broccoli (frozen, microwaved broccoli is fine). If you're eating out, ask for less cheese, no margarine or butter, and double the broccoli.

29. Smoked Turkey and Cranberry Sandwich***
Spread 2 slices whole wheat bread each with 1 teaspoon reduced-fat mayonnaise. Fill with 2 slices (2 ounces) smoked turkey sliced for sandwiches (check label for no more than 2 grams of fat per ounce), 2 tablespoons cranberry sauce, and a piece of romaine lettuce. Serve with 1 cup sliced celery sticks. Have an apple for dessert.

30. Turkey/Avocado/Bacon Wrap
On an 8- or 9-inch tortilla (preferably whole wheat), place 2 slices (2 ounces) turkey breast sliced for sandwiches (check label for no more than 2 grams of fat per ounce), 1 strip bacon, crumbled (save time by microwaving precooked bacon such as Oscar Mayer Ready-to-Serve Bacon), 2 tablespoons diced avocado, and 2 slices tomato (optional: 1 tablespoon salsa). Roll and serve with ½ cup baby carrots.

AFTERNOON SNACK CHOICES

You can head off the midafternoon munchies—and bolster your daily calcium intake to boot—with the snacks in this list. And you have two ways to enjoy them: Pair a Calcium Snack with a Fruit Snack (you can eat them together or separately); or choose just one of the Double Snacks, which include both a high-calcium food and a fruit. Either way, you'll be getting approximately 165 calories, 2 grams of total fat,

1 gram of saturated fat, 30 grams of carbohydrates, 8 grams of protein, 9 milligrams of cholesterol, 94 milligrams of sodium, 2 grams of fiber, and 267 milligrams of calcium.

You're welcome to come up with your own snack combinations, too. Simply apply these key nutrition guidelines.

- Aim for 165 calories.
- Include 2 servings of fruit (one serving equals ½ cup cut-up fruit or berries, one small piece of fruit, or ¾ cup citrus juice).
- Also include 1 cup of milk, yogurt, or calcium-fortified soy milk, or 1 ounce of reduced-fat cheese.

Calcium Snacks
If you pick an item from this list, remember to pair it with one of the Fruit Snacks.

1. Classic Refresher
Drink 1 cup (a half-pint carton) of chilled nonfat milk.

2. Vegetarian Refresher
Drink 1 cup or an 8–9 ounce box of chilled vanilla or other flavored, low-fat, calcium-fortified soy milk (for convenience, get Edensoy Extra Original 8.45-ounce cartons).

3. Yogurt Your Way
Have 1 cup (8 ounces) nonfat yogurt in your choice of flavors (check label for about 120 calories per cup).

4. Maple Milk
Heat 1 cup nonfat milk or low-fat, calcium-fortified vanilla soy milk; stir in 1 teaspoon maple syrup.

5. Almond Milk
Add a few drops almond extract to 1 cup nonfat milk or low-fat, calcium-fortified vanilla soy milk, cold or heated.

6. Café au Lait
Mix together 1 cup hot brewed or instant coffee (regular or decaf) and 1 cup hot nonfat milk or low-fat, calcium-fortified vanilla soy milk plus 1 teaspoon sugar, if desired.

7. Iced Café au Lait
Mix together 1 cup cold nonfat milk or low-fat, calcium-fortified plain soy milk with 1 cup room-temperature brewed coffee. Add ice and 1 teaspoon sugar if desired.

8. Cheese and a Pickle** ***
Have 2 individually wrapped wedges of spreadable Laughing Cow Light—we like the French Onion and Garlic & Herb varieties—or 70 calories' worth of other cheese on 2 Reduced Fat Triscuits (or 33 calories' worth of another whole grain cracker) with a pickle of your choice.

9. Cheese and a Crunch**
Have 1½ slices (1½ ounces) reduced-fat American cheese (check label for no more that 5 grams fat per slice, such as Borden's 2% American cheese singles) wrapped around a stick of celery. (Optional: Dip in hot and spicy mustard.)

10. Hot Chocolate
Heat 1 cup nonfat milk. Add ½ tablespoon chocolate syrup such as Hershey's. (Optional: Add a few drops vanilla extract and top with 2 tablespoons canned whipped cream.)

11. Chocolate Milk
Mix 1 cup cold nonfat milk or low-fat, calcium-fortified plain or vanilla soy milk with ½ tablespoon chocolate syrup such as Hershey's.

12. Strawberry Milk

Mix 1 cup cold nonfat milk or low-fat, calcium-fortified plain or vanilla soy milk with 2 teaspoons strawberry powder such as Nesquik.

Fruit Snacks

Combine any of the items in this list with one of the Calcium Snacks.

13. Just Fruit

Have 1 apple, pear, orange, peach, small banana, or other piece of fruit of your choice.

14. Just Berries

Have ½ to 1 cup berries, such as strawberries, raspberries, or blueberries, fresh or frozen (unsweetened).

15. Fruit to Go

Have ½ cup (a 4-ounce container) of fruit canned in its own juice (not syrup). Check labels for around 60 calories per serving. For convenience, use single-serving, peel-top containers, such as Del Monte Fruit Naturals Sliced Peaches in Pear and Peach Juice or Dole Pineapple FruitBowls.

16. Frozen Grapes

Put a cluster of grapes about the size of your fist (½ cup) in the freezer for several hours. Enjoy.

17. Just for You, Baby

Tuck into a jar of baby-food peaches or other baby-food fruit (check label for no more than 70 calories per serving).

18. Apricot Indulgence

Have 3 dried apricots (or 6 halves). As rich and sweet as candy!

19. Ready Raisins

Grab a pack of Sun-Maid's handy ½-ounce minipacks of raisins. A 2-tablespoon serving of raisins is already measured for you.

20. Applesauce Comfort

Applesauce makes a great snack because it feels like comfort food. Try convenient single-serving, peel-top containers with ½ cup applesauce (such as Mott's Natural Style Apple Sauce or Mott's Healthy Harvest—any flavor).

21. Tangy Thirst Quencher

Drink a 6-ounce can of grapefruit juice.

22. Luscious Dried Plums

Enjoy 3 succulent pitted dried plums (that's the sexy new name for prunes!). We like the Sunsweet orange essence flavored ones.

23. Portable Fruit Cocktail

Have ½ cup (4 ounces) fruit cocktail canned in juice (no syrup). For convenience, use the single-serving, peel-top containers, such as Del Monte Fruit Naturals Chunky Mixed Fruits in Fruit Juices.

24. Make It Melon

You can have ¼ of a medium cantaloupe, ⅛ of a medium honeydew, or 1 cup watermelon, canteloupe, or honeydew pieces.

Double Snacks

Each of the following items combines a fruit with a calcium-rich food for a complete snack. If you eat it in the afternoon, you won't feel ravenous by dinnertime.

25. Peach Slush

In a blender, combine 1 cup (8 ounces) peach-flavored nonfat yogurt (check labels for about 120 calories per cup) with a peeled and sliced, ripe peach or ½ cup canned peach (in juice, not syrup). Add 1 or 2 ice cubes and blend until smooth. (For variety, make slush with berry-flavored yogurt and fresh or frozen, unsweetened berries.)

26. Strawberry Soy Milk Smoothie
In a blender, combine until smooth 1 cup low-fat, calcium-fortified vanilla soy milk, half of a ripe banana, and ¼ cup strawberries (fresh or frozen, unsweetened). (Alternative: Use 1 cup nonfat milk.)

27. Fruit and Cheese**
Slice a ripe pear or apple; eat with 1 ounce room-temperature reduced-fat Cheddar. Pick a brand like Kraft 2% Milk Sharp Cheddar or Cabot Light Vermont Cheddar 50% with about 5 grams fat per ounce (the lower-fat brands just don't cut it with fruit).

28. Fruit Blast Yogurt
Mix ½ cup fresh or frozen, unsweetened blueberries or strawberries or any chopped fruit with 1 cup (8 ounces) nonfat berry-flavored yogurt (check label for about 120 calories per cup).

29. Banana Smoothie
In a blender, combine until smooth: ½ cup nonfat milk, half of a ripe banana, and ½ cup (4 ounces) nonfat vanilla-flavored yogurt (check label for about 120 calories per cup). Blend in 1 or 2 ice cubes and a few drops vanilla extract.

30. Tropical Yogurt
Stir 2 tablespoons tropical dried fruit mix into 1 cup (8 ounces) nonfat pineapple- or apricot-flavored yogurt (check label for no more than 120 calories per cup). Mix in a few drops coconut extract.

DINNER CHOICES

The meals in this list should convince you that healthy dinners can be fast and easy. Some of the items require no cooking; others, only the shortest amount of preparation time.
What if you're planning to eat out? We've got you covered
there, too, with nutritious choices from some of the most
popular chain restaurants. The average dinner supplies 390
calories, 10 grams of total fat, 3 grams of saturated fat, 50
grams of carbohydrates, 25 grams of protein, 74 milligrams
of cholesterol, 845 milligrams of sodium, 8 grams of fiber,
and 217 milligrams of calcium.

Of course, you should feel free to improvise your own dinner menu from ingredients you already have on hand. Ideally,
your meal will meet the following nutrition requirements.

- It supplies about 390 calories.
- It allows for two servings of vegetables (one serving
  equals 1 cup of raw leafy greens; ½ cup of other vegetables,
  cooked or raw; or ¾ cup of tomato or vegetable juice).

Effortless Home Cooking
Sometimes you want the comfort of dinner at home, but you
don't want the fuss. You *really* don't! For those occasions,
you'll love these hassle-free meals.

I. Lentil Soup and French Bread***
Heat 1½ cups lentil soup (for example, approximately ¾
of a 19-ounce can Progresso Classics Lentil Soup). Serve
with a large slice (about 6 inches long) of warm French
bread (for example, ⅙ of Pillsbury's Crusty French Loaf,
found in refrigerated cans) spread with 1 tablespoon diet
margarine (such as Smart Beat Super Light or I Can't Believe It's Not Butter Light). Serve with ½ cup of red pepper strips.

2. Pizza!** ***

Have 1 slice of a large (14-inch) pizza or 1½ slices of a medium (12-inch) pizza topped with two vegetables, such as mushrooms and green pepper. Use only medium- or thin-crust pizza (such as Domino's Hand-Tossed Pizza). For frozen pizza, check labels, and have 265–280 calories' worth. Serve with a salad: 1 cup mixed greens, ½ cup chopped vegetable of your choice, such as tomatoes, peppers, carrots, etc., with 2 tablespoons reduced-calorie dressing.

3. Chicken and Veggies

Microwave according to package directions Smart Ones Spicy Szechuan-Style Vegetables and Chicken or similar frozen meal (check labels for about 270–280 calories, 4–7 grams fat). Serve with ¾ cup raw veggies—red pepper strips and cucumber sticks would be nice—and 1 cup nonfat milk.

4. Breakfast for Dinner

Make 2 eggs your way: poached, soft-boiled, or scrambled in a nonstick pan sprayed with butter-flavored Pam. Serve with 2 slices whole wheat toast with 2 teaspoons jam or jelly on each. Add a 6-ounce glass of tomato juice.

5. Tortellini, Manicotti, or Lasagna** ***

Microwave according to package directions Healthy Choice Bowls Cheese Tortellini, Healthy Choice Manicotti with Three Cheeses, or similar frozen meal (check label for 300–330 calories, 9–12 grams fat). Add a salad made of 1 cup romaine lettuce or mixed greens, ½ cup chopped vegetables of your choice (such as tomato or cucumber) tossed with 1½ tablespoons reduced-calorie salad dressing.

6. Veggie Burger on the Ranch***

Microwave or grill a vegetable burger according to package directions. Choose patties in the 110–130 calorie range (such as The Original Gardenburger or Amy's California Veggie Burger). Place on a whole grain bun spread with 1 tablespoon reduced-calorie ranch (or Caesar) dressing. (Optional: Instead of dressing, use mustard and ketchup to taste.) Add 2 thick slices tomato and 2 slices romaine lettuce. Serve with ½ cup raw veggies (like carrot and celery sticks) and ⅓ cup baked beans.

7. Amy's Skillet Meal Pasta and Vegetables Alfredo**
Serves 2
Add contents of package along with 1 cup chopped broccoli (fresh or frozen) to a nonstick skillet sprayed with Pam. Cook according to package directions. At the last minute, stir in ½ cup cooked skinless chicken strips (such as Perdue Short Cuts or Louis Rich Carving Board). Eat half for one serving.

8. Cereal for Dinner
Put 1 cup raisin bran in a big bowl, add 2 teaspoons roasted sunflower or pumpkin seeds and 1 chopped apple, and top with 1 cup nonfat milk.

9. Beef and Veggies**
Microwave according to package directions Uncle Ben's Spicy Beef and Broccoli Bowl, Lean Cuisine Southern Beef Tips, or similar frozen meal (check label for 270–300 calories, 5–9 grams fat). Add a salad: 1 cup romaine lettuce or mixed greens (save time with prewashed, bagged greens) and ½ cup cherry tomatoes or other vegetable of your choice. Dress with 1 tablespoon regular dressing or 2 tablespoons reduced calorie.

10. Tomato Soup and Grilled Cheese** ***
Heat 1 to 1½ cups tomato soup (check labels because brands vary in calories; have about 85 calories' worth). Grilled cheese sandwich: Spread 2 slices whole wheat bread with 1 teaspoon diet margarine (such as Smart

Beat Super Light or I Can't Believe It's Not Butter Light) each. With buttered sides out, place 2 slices (2 ounces) reduced-fat cheese (less than 5 grams of fat per slice, such as Borden's 2% American cheese singles or Cabot Light Vermont Cheddar 50% Singles) between bread slices. Grill in a nonstick pan sprayed with Pam or in a toaster oven until cheese melts.

11. Vegetarian Chili with Cornbread***
Heat 1 cup canned vegetarian chili. Serve with a 2-inch by 3-inch piece of cornbread (about 1.5 ounces; check your supermarket bakery department) or one Pillsbury Cornbread Twist (in refrigerated cans).

12. Fettuccine Alfredo
Microwave according to package directions Lean Cuisine Everyday Favorites Chicken Fettucine or similar frozen meal (check label for 270–280 calories, 6–10 grams fat). Steam or microwave 1 cup fresh or frozen broccoli. Transfer to plate. Pour chicken fettuccine over broccoli. Serve with a 4-ounce glass of wine.

13. Seafood Dinner
Microwave according to package directions Lean Cuisine Baked Fish, Healthy Choice Lemon Pepper Fish, or similar frozen meal (check label for 290–320 calories, 6–8 grams fat). Add 1 cup steamed or microwaved vegetables, fresh or frozen, tossed with a spritz of lemon juice and 1 teaspoon olive oil.

14. Chicken and Baked Beans
Dark meat lovers: Have a thigh, no skin. White meat lovers: Have 2 ounces skinless breast (about two-thirds of a deck of cards). To save time, go with rotisserie chicken from the supermarket. Add ¾ cup canned baked beans, heated, and 1 cup microwaved or steamed matchstick-cut carrots.

Only a Little Cooking Required

We mean it when we say these meals call for minimal cooking—boiling pasta or microwaving asparagus, for example. But we bet you'll love the results!

15. Waffles Florentine** ***
Serves 2 (2 waffles each)

Toast 4 whole grain frozen waffles (check label for about 180 calories for 2 waffles) and microwave a microwave-ready 9-ounce bag of fresh baby spinach such as Ready Pac brand (or 2 cups frozen chopped spinach) according to package directions (about 3 minutes). Fry 4 eggs in a nonstick skillet sprayed with Pam. Top each waffle with 1 egg and ¼ of the spinach (about ½ cup) and 1 tablespoon grated Parmesan cheese.

16. Southwestern Beans, Rice, and Cheese**
Serves 2

Microwave one Cascadian Farm Aztec Organic Vegetarian Meal (a frozen medley of black beans, brown rice, corn, red peppers, wheat berries, garlic, and spices) according to package directions; set aside, covered. Microwave a microwave-ready 9-ounce bag of fresh baby spinach such as Ready Pac brand (or 2 cups frozen chopped spinach) according to package directions (about 3 minutes). Add cooked spinach to beans and rice. Divide mixture between 2 plates. (For men following the Ice Cream Diet, add a heaping ⅓ cup cooked chicken strips such as Perdue Short Cuts or Louis Rich Carving Board.) Top each plate with 4 tablespoons Parmesan cheese and microwave for 1 minute to melt cheese. Have 1 cup canteloupe cubes for dessert.

17. Four-Minute Parmesan Spinach with Salmon**
Serves 2

Microwave a microwave-ready 9-ounce bag of fresh spinach such as Ready Pac brand (or 2 cups frozen chopped spinach) according to package directions (about 3 minutes). Carefully remove hot spinach from bag and fork out 1 cup in each of 2 microwave-safe bowls. In each bowl add ⅓ heaping cup salmon from uneaten portion you brought home from a restaurant meal such as #26 (alternate: use ⅓ cup cooked chicken strips like Perdue Short Cuts or Louis Rich Carving Board) and sprinkle on 3 tablespoons Parmesan cheese. Microwave each bowl for 30–45 seconds, until cheese begins to melt. Add 1 slice whole wheat bread and a 4-ounce glass of wine.

18. Elegant Salmon, Couscous, and Asparagus
Serves 2

In a small 1½-quart baking dish, pour 1 cup white wine and 1 cup water. Add 5 peppercorns, a whole clove, 2 bay leaves, and a peeled clove of garlic. Put in the oven at 350°F. When it comes to a simmer, add two 3-ounce pieces of boneless salmon fillet. Cook skin-side down for 8 minutes or until just done all the way through. With a slotted spoon, remove salmon from liquid. Serve each piece of salmon with 1 cup whole wheat couscous (made according to package directions starting with ½ cup dry couscous for 2 servings, as in Fantastic brand) and 1 cup steamed or microwaved asparagus with a spritz of lemon.

19. Broccoli Pasta with Shrimp
Serves 2

In a medium pot, cook according to package directions 1⅓ cups dry whole wheat pasta (ziti, penne, or other short pasta). While pasta is cooking, in a large nonstick skillet over medium heat, add 1 tablespoon olive or canola oil and a clove of minced garlic (or 1 teaspoon garlic powder). Sauté garlic for 30 seconds, then add about 15 large or 24 medium peeled shrimp (5 ounces), either fresh or frozen and thawed. Cook until shrimp turn pink, about 4–5 minutes, stirring constantly. Remove shrimp and garlic, add 1 teaspoon olive oil, and sauté 1½ cups fresh or frozen chopped broccoli until tender. Drain pasta when done. Mix with broccoli. Serve half of the broccoli-pasta mixture with half of the shrimp.

20. Zucchini and Chicken Pasta
Serves 2
Boil 1⅓ cups dry whole wheat pasta (ziti, penne, or other short pasta). In the 11 minutes or so it takes to boil, heat 1 cup meatless spaghetti sauce (check labels for no more than 3 grams fat per ½ cup) and set aside ⅔ cup (4 ounces) precooked, skinless chicken strips (try Perdue Short Cuts or Louis Rich Carving Board). Also, chop 1 cup zucchini and place in colander. You can "cook" the zucchini by pouring the hot pasta water over it when you drain the cooked pasta into the colander. Mix all ingredients together, divide in two, and serve.

Eating Out
An eating plan just isn't complete if it doesn't allow for the occasional dinner out. Happily, we've found lots of ways you can enjoy restaurant food—without expanding your waistline!

21. Spaghetti with Red Sauce and Seafood
At Olive Garden, order Shrimp Primavera; have half, take the rest home. In other restaurants, have a cup of spaghetti with about ½ cup tomato sauce and 2 ounces seafood—about 10 large shrimp, 8 mussels, or 6 clams. At Olive Garden or elsewhere, add a side salad (1 cup mixed greens); use 1 tablespoon of reduced-calorie dressing.

22. Olive Garden Chicken Giardino
This dish features vegetables and chicken tossed with pasta in a lemon-herb sauce. Leave about ⅕ on your plate. Entrée comes with a side salad; use 1 tablespoon reduced-calorie dressing.

23. A Taste of Greece or the Middle East
Order chicken and vegetable kabob. Have all the skewered vegetables and about 2½ ounces chicken (usually about one-third of the total chicken). Take leftover chicken home. Have a side Greek salad (at least 1 cup of

greens without the feta cheese—order dressing on the side and use 1 tablespoon) plus 1 cup rice.

24. A Taste of China***
Order beef and broccoli; chicken and broccoli; or shrimp and broccoli. Or these same dishes with mixed vegetables instead of broccoli. Your strategy: Ask for more vegetables than beef, chicken, or shrimp, and ask them to stir-fry in very little oil. Have 1¼ cup entrée with ¾ cup steamed rice. If they won't accommodate your requests for less oil, more veggies, etc., then just have 1 cup entrée and ¾ cup steamed rice.

25. Boston Market Chicken Dinner
Order a Quarter Dark Meat Chicken (ask for no skin) or a Quarter White Meat Chicken (ask for no skin or wing). Have a side of Garlic Dill New Potatoes (¾ cup). Add a side of Steamed Vegetable Medley or Herbed Sweet Corn (ask for a heaping serving, about a cup). Skip the Cornbread that comes with your meal.

26. Grilled Salmon**
At TGI Friday's, order the Jack Daniel's Salmon (tell your waiter not to bring extra sauce). Have a piece of salmon no bigger than a deck of cards. Take the rest home. This comes with chef's vegetables; request that they be cooked in minimal oil. Also, ask for your baked potato plain, and have half. Use the same strategy when ordering salmon in other restaurants.

27. Dinner at the Mall***
At Au Bon Pain have half the huge Fields 'n Feta Wrap (split one order with a friend), plus a medium serving (12 ounces) of Garden Vegetable Soup, or another non-creamed vegetable soup.

28. Another Dinner at the Mall***
At Schlotzsky's Deli have the small-size Chicken Dijon sandwich from the "Light and Flavorful" menu plus a small Garden Salad with a tablespoon of Light Italian dressing (no more than ⅓ packet, or 1 tablespoon).

29. A Stop at Wendy's***
Have the large-size chili. Order the side salad; use ⅓ of a packet fat-free French dressing.

30. Mac and Cheese at the Diner**
Ask for an order of mac and cheese (have 1 cup) plus order 2 side vegetables (such as broccoli and carrots). Try them all served on the same plate so you can mix them up in a cheesy pasta medley.

CHAPTER TEN

Mix-and-Match
Menus for Men

Men love ice cream every bit as much as women do. When Brian Wansink, Ph.D., a University of Illinois marketing professor, asked more than 1,000 people to name their favorite comfort food, both genders made ice cream their overwhelming number-one choice. So if you're a guy, rest assured: This is *your* diet, too.

We've designed slightly different menus for you because as a man, you need more calories than a woman does—lucky you! In the following pages, you'll find at least 30 menu options each for breakfast, lunch, dinner, and an afternoon snack. That's more than *four million* possible meal combinations, which means any hungry man should be able to custom-tailor this diet to suit his appetite and lifestyle. Incidentally, your choices include very guy-friendly fare like fast-food burgers, pizza, and dinners that come out of a can or the freezer.

Following the Ice Cream Diet gets even easier. All you need to do is pick one breakfast, one lunch, one snack, and one dinner every day. Together, your choices will provide about 1,625 calories, leaving room for a cool, creamy 1½-cup serving of ice cream or frozen yogurt—375 calories' worth—as a nightcap. All told, you'll be getting 2,000 calories a day, an intake that should help the average man lose well over a pound in a week, or up to 50 pounds in a year.

If you want to slim down, don't forget about physical activity. It's a must. In fact, once you reach your goal weight, you need to keep on exercising to stay there. Data from successful dieters proves it! You'll learn more about the exercise component of the Ice Cream Diet in part V.

SMART EATING MADE EASY

We've tried to coordinate the men's and women's menus as much as possible, so you and your partner can follow the Ice Cream Diet together. While you have many meals and snacks to choose from, you should feel free to enjoy your favorites as often as you like. It's satisfying, and it's sensible, too. After all, you want to use up the ingredients that you're buying.

Do try to avoid eating the same foods every day, however. The more variety you build into your diet, the more nutrients you'll be feeding your body. And good nutrition is the cornerstone of the Ice Cream Diet.

No matter how you mix and match your menu options, you'll be getting about 22 percent of your daily calories from fat, and about 7 percent from saturated fat. These numbers are consistent with National Institutes of Health guidelines for maintaining a healthy cholesterol profile and minimizing heart disease risk. We have included some items with slightly higher saturated fat contents; they're marked with two asterisks (**). Enjoying these foods on occasion is fine; they will balance out with the other choices that are quite low in saturated fat. But you should avoid making a

---

IF YOU PREFER SOY MILK

In any meal that calls for nonfat milk, you may substitute soy milk. Choose a product that supplies up to 110 calories per cup and supplies at least 30 percent of the Daily Value, or 300 milligrams, of calcium per cup.

ESTIMATING PORTIONS

The following comparisons can come in handy when measuring cups and spoons aren't available.

• A half-cup looks like a tennis ball, or about half of a man's tightly balled fist.

• A tablespoon looks like half of a Ping-Pong ball, or about half of a man's thumb.

• A teaspoon looks a little smaller than the tip of a man's thumb.

---

steady diet of them, as they'll take you over the 7 percent saturated fat limit.

Also important for heart health is watching your sodium intake, especially if you have high blood pressure. On the Ice Cream Diet, the average daily intake is slightly higher than the 2,400 milligrams recommended by the American Heart Association. That's largely because we've included a number of convenience foods among our menu options. You can limit your sodium consumption further by choosing meals with three asterisks (***) sparingly, as their sodium is on the high side. And when these items call for convenience products like tomato juice, V8, or pasta sauce, stick with the reduced-sodium or low-sodium versions.

MAN-SIZED BENEFITS

Just like the women's version of the Ice Cream Diet, the men's version provides for at least eight nutrient-packed servings of fruits and vegetables a day. For guys, produce has a bonus health benefit. Certain kinds—like apples, onions, garlic, and broccoli—are naturally rich in quercetin, an antioxidant that appears to relieve prostatitis, or a painfully inflamed prostate.

In one preliminary study, researchers at the Harbor–UCLA Medical Center in Torrance, California, gave 15 men with chronic prostatitis 500 milligrams of quercetin twice a day for 1 month. Two-thirds of these men reported at least 25 percent improvement in their prostate pain, compared with only 20 percent of men taking placebos. Since experts have yet to determine the most effective dosage for quercetin, their advice is to keep eating quercetin-rich fruits and vegetables, which we've figured into the Ice Cream Diet.

You'll also find lots of tomato products like tomato sauce, tomato juice, and V8. All are rich in lycopene, an antioxidant that concentrates in the prostate gland and may offer protection against prostate cancer. Research suggests that eating just two to four servings of tomato sauce or tomato juice per week may cut a man's prostate cancer risk by as much as one-third.

Beyond their supplies of prostate-friendly antioxidants, fruits and vegetables contain admirable amounts of fiber. Overall, the Ice Cream Diet delivers about 28 grams of fiber a day, about twice as much as the average American male eats. That's important, because high-fiber diets appear to reduce the risk of heart attack, stroke, diabetes, and some cancers.

Fiber may offer another guy-specific benefit, too. One study found that men who ate more soluble fiber—the kind found in oatmeal, beans, and most fruits and vegetables—had lower levels of prostate-specific antigen (PSA), a major marker for prostate cancer, than men who ate less.

As you follow the Ice Cream Diet, you'll also be getting about 1,400 milligrams of bone-building calcium a day. Think men don't need milk mustaches? Then consider this: One in five people with osteoporosis is male. That may be because on average, a man's daily calcium intake amounts to less than half of the recommended 1,000 to 1,500 milligrams.

Keep in mind that as your menu choices change, all of your nutrient intakes likely will change as well—though not by much. You can mix and match meals and snacks to your heart's content, and still get the following nutrients in roughly the same amounts.

- 2,000 calories
- 49 grams of total fat (22 percent of calories)
- 15 grams of saturated fat (7 percent of calories)

- 300 grams of carbohydrates (60 percent of calories)
- 90 grams of protein (18 percent of calories)
- 288 milligrams of cholesterol
- 2,700 milligrams of sodium
- 28 grams of fiber
- 1,400 milligrams of calcium

Even though you can expect balanced nutrition from the Ice Cream Diet, I recommend taking a multivitamin/mineral supplement for extra nutritional support. For guidelines on choosing a good supplement, see "A Multi Makes Sense" on page 74. While you're there, take a moment to read "Quench Your Thirst" on page 75; it explains the importance of fluids to weight loss and overall health. Unless a menu option specifies otherwise, stick with no-calorie beverages like water, sparkling water, coffee, tea, and diet soda.

And don't forget: You're entitled to a smooth and satisfying 1½-cup, 375-calorie serving of ice cream or frozen yogurt every night. Think of it as your reward for making smart food choices the rest of the day. You just have to pick the flavor!

BREAKFAST CHOICES

To create this breakfast menu, we focused on foods that whip up fast and go down easy first thing in the morning. On average, these menu options deliver 430 calories, 8 grams of total fat, 2 grams of saturated fat, 71 grams of carbohydrates, 18 grams of protein, 35 milligrams of cholesterol, 440 milligrams of sodium, 9 grams of fiber, and 397 milligrams of calcium.

For the cereal-based breakfasts, you can pour all the milk into your bowl, or you can save some to wash down your meal or to add to coffee or tea. Likewise, the milk in noncereal breakfasts can be consumed "as is" or mixed into coffee (as in a latte) or tea. When a menu option calls for yogurt, choose a nonfat variety that has about 120 calories per cup, like Dannon Light 'n Fit.

We hope that you'll find many breakfasts that suit your appetite and lifestyle. But you're always welcome to design your own morning meals. Ideally, they'll meet these basic nutritional guidelines.

- Aim for no more than 430 calories.
- Aim for two servings of fruit (one serving equals ½ cup cut-up fruit or berries, one small piece of fruit, or ¾ cup citrus juice).
- Include 1 cup of milk, yogurt, or calcium-fortified soy milk, or 1 ounce of reduced-fat cheese.

1. Cinnamon Apple Oatmeal

Cook ½ cup dry oatmeal—quick cooking, old fashioned, or instant—in ½ cup nonfat milk, ½ cup water according to package directions (usually about 1–2 minutes in microwave oven). Top with (or cook with) a medium chopped apple, a dash of cinnamon, and 2 tablespoons raisins. Serve with 2 teaspoons maple syrup or honey, and 1 cup nonfat milk.

2. Bagel and Cream Cheese***

Spread a 2.5-ounce to 3-ounce bagel (for example, Lender's Refrigerated Honey Wheat Bagels are 2.85 ounces) with 2 tablespoons reduced-fat cream cheese. Serve with 1 cup nonfat milk, 1 cup fruit salad.

3. Peanut Butter Toast

Toast 2 slices whole wheat bread and spread each with 2 teaspoons peanut butter (optional: use almond butter) and 2 teaspoons jam. Serve with 1 cup fruit of your choice and 1 cup nonfat milk.

4. Strawberry Slush

In a blender, combine 1 cup (8 ounces) nonfat strawberry-flavored yogurt (no more than 120 calories), ½ cup strawberries (fresh or frozen, unsweetened), 1 teaspoon honey, a medium ripe banana, and several ice cubes (add cubes one at a time). Serve with 9 Reduced Fat Triscuits (or 146 calories' worth of another whole grain cracker).

5. On-the-Go Breakfast
Pack 1 can Slim-Fast (11 ounces, any flavor) or other meal replacement drink at about 220 calories per can. Take along a small banana and 2 tablespoons raisins (for example, a small, ½-ounce packet of Sun-Maid raisins), and 4 Reduced Fat Triscuits (or 65 calories' worth of another whole grain cracker).

6. English Muffin and Fruit**
Toast a whole wheat or oat bran English muffin. Spread one half with 1 teaspoon butter or trans-free margarine, the other with 1 teaspoon jam or jelly. Serve with 1 cup nonfat milk, 1 cup cantaloupe pieces, and 6 ounces orange juice.

7. Bran Flakes with Blueberries***
Use 1 cup flaky bran cereal (with about 130 calories and 7 grams fiber, like Post Bran Flakes) with 1 teaspoon sugar, 1 cup fresh or frozen, unsweetened blueberries, and 1 cup nonfat milk. Serve with a slice of whole wheat toast spread with 1 teaspoon butter or trans-free margarine and a teaspoon of jam.

8. Waffles and Strawberries***
Prepare 2 toaster waffles, preferably whole grain (check label for no more than 170 calories per 2 waffles, as in Eggo Nutri-Grain). Spread each with a teaspoon of diet margarine (such as Smart Beat Super Light or I Can't Believe It's Not Butter Light). Top each with 2 teaspoons maple syrup and ½ cup fresh or frozen (unsweetened and thawed) strawberries, smashed. Serve with 1 cup nonfat milk.

9. Hot Chocolate and Toast***
Have 1 mug hot chocolate (1 cup nonfat milk, heated, mixed with 1 tablespoon Hershey's syrup). Serve with

2 slices whole wheat toast each spread with 1 teaspoon diet margarine (such as Smart Beat Super Light or I Can't Believe It's Not Butter Light) and 1 teaspoon jam or jelly, plus 1 cup fresh or frozen, unsweetened raspberries or other berries.

10. In-the-Car Breakfast** ***
Pack 6 Wasa crisp bread slices (or 180 calories and 12 grams fiber's worth of another whole rye cracker) with 2 part-skim mozzarella cheese sticks (such as Sargento 24-g String Cheese Snacks, which come in a six-pack), a 6.75-ounce orange juice box (such as Minute Maid), and 2 tablespoons raisins (for example, a small, ½-ounce packet of Sun-Maid raisins).

11. Bran Muffin and Applesauce
Have a medium bran muffin (3 ounces, about the size of a tennis ball) with 1 cup nonfat milk, an orange, and ½ cup unsweetened applesauce (for example, a single-serving, peel-top container of Mott's Natural Style Apple Sauce).

12. Shredded Wheat and Strawberries***
Top 1½ cups shredded wheat (for example, Post bite-size Shredded Wheat 'N Bran or other cereal containing about 160 calories per cup) with 1 cup fresh or frozen, unsweetened strawberries and 1 cup nonfat milk.

13. At-Your-Desk Breakfast
Have 1 cereal bar (no more than 150 calories, such as Kellogg's NutriGrain bar), ½-pint container nonfat milk, a small apple, and a zip-top snack bag containing 3 dried apricots (or 6 halves) and 8 almonds.

14. Apple Yogurt
Top 1 cup (8 ounces) nonfat fruit-flavored yogurt (no more than 120 calories) with 1 medium chopped apple and 2 tablespoons raisins. Serve with 10 Reduced Fat Triscuits (or 163 calories' worth of another whole grain cracker).

15. Muesli and Apples

Top ¾ cup muesli (such as Kellogg's Mueslix or other mueslis at about 150 calories per half-cup) with a medium chopped apple and 1 cup nonfat milk. Serve with a tangerine.

16. French Toast and Berries***

Dip 2 slices whole wheat bread in ⅓ cup Egg Beaters or 2 beaten egg whites mixed with 2 tablespoons nonfat milk. Brown in nonstick skillet sprayed with Pam. Top each slice with 1½ teaspoons maple syrup. Serve with 1 cup fresh or frozen, unsweetened blueberries and 1 cup nonfat milk.

17. English Muffin and Peanut Butter

Toast 1 oat bran or whole wheat English muffin and spread with 2 teaspoons peanut butter and 2 teaspoons jam. Serve with 1 cup nonfat milk, 1 orange, and ½ cup unsweetened applesauce.

18. Raisin Bran and Banana***

Top 1 cup raisin bran (for example, Post, Kellogg's, or any other brand that's about 140 calories for ¾ cup) with a medium sliced banana, 2 tablespoons sliced or chopped almonds, and 1 cup nonfat milk.

19. Cheese Toast***

In toaster oven heat 2 slices whole wheat bread each topped with 1 slice (1 ounce) of reduced-fat cheese (check label for no more than 5 grams fat per ounce, such as Borden's 2% American cheese singles or Cabot Light Vermont Cheddar 50% Singles). Serve with ¾ cup (6 ounces) orange juice and 3 dried apricots (or 6 halves).

20. Peanut Butter Crackers and Fruit

Spread 1 tablespoon peanut butter and 1 tablespoon jam of your choice on 130 calories' worth of whole wheat or rye crackers such as 8 Reduced Fat Triscuits or 4 slices rye crisp bread (such as Wasa). Serve with 1 cup honey-dew melon pieces and 1 cup nonfat milk.

21. Bagel, Lox, and Cream Cheese***
Spread a 2.5- to 3-ounce bagel (for example, Lender's Refrigerated Honey Wheat Bagels, 2.85 ounces each) with 2 tablespoons reduced-fat cream cheese and top with 1 ounce smoked salmon (about 1–2 strips). Serve with 1 cup fresh or frozen (unsweetened and thawed) straw-berries and 1 cup nonfat milk.

22. Cheerios and Blueberries***
Top 1½ cups Cheerios (or 165 calories' worth of other whole grain "O"-type cereal) with 1 cup fresh or frozen, unsweetened blueberries and 1 cup nonfat milk. Serve with a small banana.

23. Toast and Eggs** ***
Scramble 2 medium eggs in a nonstick skillet sprayed with Pam. (Optional: Scramble with ¼ cup mushrooms and 1 teaspoon chopped scallion.) Serve with a slice of whole wheat toast spread with 1 teaspoon butter or trans-free margarine. Serve with 1 cup fruit salad and 1 cup nonfat milk.

24. Cheese Grits**
Stir 4 tablespoons (1 ounce) shredded, reduced-fat cheese (such as Kraft 2% Milk Sharp Cheddar or Cabot Light Vermont Cheddar 50%) into 1 cup hot grits cooked ac-cording to package directions. Serve with half of a large grapefruit, 1 medium apple, and 1 cup nonfat milk.

25. Breakfast Burrito***
Scramble ½ cup Egg Beaters (or 1 egg and 1 egg white) in a nonstick skillet with 1 teaspoon butter or trans-free margarine. Place in a warmed, 8-inch tortilla (preferably whole wheat, such as Cedarlane brand) with 2 table-spoons salsa, roll, and eat. Serve with 1 cup of nonfat milk and an orange.

26. Waffles with Maple Syrup***

Top each of 2 toasted frozen waffles, preferably whole grain (check labels for no more than 170 calories for 2 waffles such as Eggo Nutri-Grain) with 1 teaspoon butter or trans-free margarine and 1 teaspoon maple syrup. Serve with 1 cup cantaloupe or honeydew chunks and 1 cup of nonfat milk.

27. Hot Cereal with Apricots

Microwave ½ cup multigrain hot cereal (for example, Quaker, Mother's, or any other brand that's about 130 calories per half-cup uncooked). Use package directions, but instead of using all water, use half water and half milk; in most cases that means ½ cup water and ½ cup milk to ½ cup dry cereal. Cook with 3 dried apricots (or 6 halves), chopped. (It usually takes 1–2 minutes.) Serve with ½ cup nonfat milk and ½ cup unsweetened applesauce. Add 1 slice whole wheat toast spread with a teaspoon of butter or trans-free margarine.

28. Cinnamon Toast***

Toast 2 slices whole wheat bread. Spread each with 1 teaspoon butter or trans-free margarine, ½ teaspoon sugar, and a sprinkling of cinnamon. Serve with 1 cup nonfat milk and a medium apple.

29. Fiber Power Breakfast

Top ½ cup high-fiber cereal (serving size may vary from ⅓ to ¾ cup; look for cereal with about 10–13 grams of fiber per serving, such as Kellogg's All Bran, General Foods' Fiber One, or Kellogg's Bran Buds) with ¼ cup low-fat granola, a small chopped apple, and 1 cup nonfat milk. Serve with ¾ cup orange juice.

30. Breakfast at the Diner***

Order a toasted English muffin and 2 eggs—soft boiled, poached, or scrambled in very little oil (doesn't hurt to ask!). Also order a cup of nonfat milk and a cup of fruit salad.

LUNCH CHOICES

Lunchtime can be a dietary danger zone, especially if you're eating at work or on the go. We've come up with some menu options for any situation—even those rare occasions when you can eat at home! No matter which meal you choose, you'll be getting about 465 calories, 12 grams of total fat, 4 grams of saturated fat, 66 grams of carbohydrates, 23 grams of protein; 48 milligrams of cholesterol, 920 milligrams of sodium; 8 grams of fiber, and 218 milligrams of calcium.

To meet your body's nutritional requirements, any lunch of your creation should include the following:

- No more than 465 calories
- Two servings of vegetables (one serving equals 1 cup of raw leafy greens; ½ cup of other vegetables, cooked or raw; or ¾ cup of tomato or vegetable juice)

Lunch on the Job

Many of the following menu options are ideal for brown-bagging. If you don't have time to pack your lunch, you can always stop at the supermarket and pick up one of the frozen entrées suggested here. They couldn't be more convenient. And they taste great! If you haven't tried "TV dinners" lately, you just might be surprised by how much they've improved.

1. Tupperware Tuna, Bean, and Corn Salad

In a plastic container with a lid, combine half of a 6-ounce can of drained, water-packed tuna with ⅓ cup rinsed canned beans (garbanzo or cannellini beans are good choices here) and ½ cup canned or frozen corn. Add ½ cup halved cherry tomatoes and ½ cup chopped green or red pepper. Toss with 1½ tablespoons Italian dressing. Optional: Add 1–2 tablespoons fresh parsley, basil, or dill.

2. Chicken Enchilada

Microwave according to package directions Lean Cuisine Chicken Enchilada Suiza with Mexican-Style Rice or Smart Ones Chicken Enchilada Suiza, or similar frozen meal (check labels for about 260–280 calories, 6–9 grams fat). Serve with 1 cup cucumber slices or other vegetable of your choice. Have 1 cup grapes for dessert.

3. Ham and Cheese on Rye***

Spread 2 slices rye bread with mustard to taste. Fill sandwich with 2 slices (2 ounces) lean ham sliced for sandwiches (check label for no more than 2 grams fat per ounce) and 1 slice (1 ounce) reduced-fat cheese (less than 5 grams fat per slice, such as Borden's 2% American cheese singles or Cabot Light Vermont Cheddar 50% Singles), 3 slices tomato, and one slice romaine lettuce. Serve with ½ cup baby carrots and ⅔ cup grapes.

4. Soup and Sandwich***

Heat 1¼ cups chicken noodle, chicken rice, beef noodle, chicken gumbo, or 100 calories' worth of any other similar soup (Campbell's Ready to Serve Chicken Noodle is the perfect size). Spread 2 slices whole wheat bread with mustard to taste. Pile on 2 slices (2 ounces) turkey breast sliced for sandwiches and 2 leaves of romaine lettuce. Serve with 1 cup broccoli florets, dipped in 2 tablespoons reduced-calorie ranch dressing.

5. A Taste of Italy***

Microwave according to package directions Lean Cuisine Everyday Favorites Cheese Ravioli or similar frozen meal (check label for 260–280 calories, 6–9 grams fat). Top with 3 tablespoons grated Parmesan cheese. Add 1 cup raw vegetables of your choice. Have a peach or other fruit for dessert.

6. Bean Burrito

Microwave according to package directions Amy's Bean and Rice Burrito, Amy's Bean and Cheese Burrito, or similar frozen meal (check labels for about 260–280 calories, 6–9 grams fat). Serve with 1 cup celery sticks or other vegetable of your choice. Have an apple for dessert.

7. Roast Beef Sandwich***

Spread 2 slices whole wheat bread with 1 teaspoon each of reduced-fat mayonnaise, plus mustard to taste (horse-radish mustard tastes even better with this sandwich). Fill with 3 slices (3 ounces) lean roast beef sliced for sand-wiches (check label for no more than 2 grams fat per ounce), 4 slices tomato, and a slice of romaine lettuce. Serve with a 6-ounce can of V8.

8. Your Favorite Chicken Lunch

Microwave according to package directions a chicken-based frozen entrée such as Smart Ones Fire-Grilled Chicken and Vegetables (check label for 260–280 calories, 6–9 grams fat). Add a cup of raw vegetables of your choice and have a large apple or other fruit for dessert.

9. Tuna Salad Sandwich***

Combine 1 tablespoon reduced-fat mayonnaise and ½ teaspoon mustard with half of a 6-ounce can of tuna. Make sandwich with 2 slices whole wheat bread, 3 slices of tomato, and 2 slices romaine lettuce. Serve with a 6-ounce can V8 and 10 reduced-fat tortilla chips.

10. South of the Border

Microwave according to package directions Smart Ones Fajita Chicken Supreme, Amy's Black Bean Enchilada Whole Meal, or similar frozen meal (check label for 260–280 calories, 6–9 grams fat). Add 1 cup raw vegeta-bles of your choice. Have a banana for dessert.

11. Peanut Butter and Jelly

Make sandwich with 2 slices whole wheat bread, 2 table-spoons peanut butter, and 2 tablespoons jelly or jam. Serve with 1-cup mix of celery sticks and baby carrots.

12. Ready for Beef

Microwave according to package directions Lean Cuisine Southern Beef Tips or similar frozen meal (check label for 260–280 calories, 6–9 grams fat). Add 1 cup raw veg-etables of your choice. Have a banana for dessert.

Lunch on the Go

Think you have to give up fast-food lunches if you're trying to slim down? These menu options will change your mind!

*13. A Stop at Subway***

Order a 6-inch Subway Veggie Delite on wheat bread with extra tomato and 2 servings (4 triangles) cheese of any type and 1 tablespoon Light Mayo, Honey Mustard, or South-west dressing. (Make sure they absolutely stuff your sand-wich with vegetables—ask for extra tomatoes or peppers.) Take an apple with you for dessert. Or get a Subway Turkey Breast and Bacon Wrap, asking for an extra serving of Swiss cheese in the wrap. Order a Veggie Delite salad and use 1 tablespoon Fat-free Italian dressing. Or get a Subway Deli Tuna Sandwich ("deli" sandwiches are on smaller rolls, not subs) with a Veggie Delite salad and use 2 table-spoons Fat-free Italian dressing. Take with you a sandwich bag with ½ cup grapes or small piece of other fruit.

14. Fast Food Burgers

Order the smallest burger or cheeseburger on the menu—which usually means the "regular" size. Have mustard and ketchup; no mayonnaise. (Hamburger: Burger King, Wendy's, Hardee's or McDonald's. Cheeseburger: Wendy's or McDonald's only.) Take with you a sandwich bag with 1 cup baby carrots (or other vegetable). Take an apple or or-ange with you for dessert.

15. Grilled Chicken Sandwich

Order a Wendy's Grilled Chicken Sandwich, the KFC Tender Roast Sandwich without sauce, or the KFC Honey BBQ Sandwich. Ask for just a dab of mayonnaise or use ½ tablespoon at the most. Mustard and ketchup are fine. (Note: Chicken sandwiches at Burger King and McDonald's are too high in calories.) Take with you a sandwich bag with 1 cup red pepper slices or other vegetable. Take an apple or orange with you for dessert.

16. A Stop at Taco Bell***

Order the Taco Bell Bean Burrito or Fiesta Burrito (Beef, Chicken, or Steak). Take with you a sandwich bag of 1 cup celery and carrot sticks or other vegetable.

17. At the Salad Bar***

Take 1 cup mixed greens or romaine lettuce and 1½ cups chopped raw (plain, not marinated) vegetables of your choice (tomatoes, shredded carrots, cucumber slices, etc.), tossed with 3 tablespoons reduced-calorie dressing. Choose one of the following: ½ cup (8 tablespoons) cottage cheese, or heaping half-cup tuna (plain, no mayonnaise). Top with either 2 tablespoons chopped egg or 2 tablespoons shredded cheese and 2 tablespoons croutons. Serve with 2 slices whole wheat bread or 2 thick slices French bread (each slice about half the size of a man's palm).

18. At the Salad Bar, Vegetarian-Style

Take 1 cup mixed greens or romaine lettuce, ½ cup beans (such as garbanzo beans or pinto beans), ¼ cup plain or marinated tofu (not deep fried), and 1½ cups chopped raw (plain, not marinated) vegetables of your choice, tossed with 3 tablespoons reduced-calorie dressing. Serve with 2 slices whole wheat bread or 2 thick slices French bread (each slice about half the size of a man's palm).

19. Grilled Chicken Caesar Salad

Many restaurants use about 6 ounces chicken; you want to eat about 3 ounces, the size of a deck of cards, or about half the chicken. (Take the rest home in a doggy bag—those chicken slices will come in handy for some of the other lunches and dinners in this plan!) Eat 2 or more cups greens. Ask for dressing on the side; use 1½ tablespoons. Top with 3 tablespoons croutons (or 2 tablespoons of the really greasy type) and have either a roll (the size of a tennis ball) or a slice of bread, preferably whole wheat.

20. A Stop at Arby's***

Order the Arby's Regular Roast Beef and a Garden Salad. Use 1 tablespoon reduced-calorie Italian or reduced-calorie Buttermilk dressing.

Lunch at Home

These meals are so easy, they'll make even a novice cook feel like a master chef! And they'll satisfy just about any taste.

21. Veggie Cheeseburger

Microwave a veggie burger according to package directions. Choose patties in the 110–130 calorie range (such as The Original Gardenburger or Amy's California Veggie Burger). When nearly cooked, top burger with 1 slice (1 ounce) reduced-fat cheese (less that 5 grams fat per slice, such as Borden's 2% American cheese singles or Cabot Light Vermont Cheddar 50% Singles) and melt. Place on a whole grain bun spread with mustard and ketchup to taste. Add 3 slices tomato and 2 slices romaine lettuce. Serve with ½ cup red pepper strips or other vegetable of your choice. Have an orange for dessert.

22. Homemade Bean Burrito

Top a warmed 8-inch tortilla (whole wheat is best, such as Cedarlane brand) with ⅓ cup canned pinto or black beans, partly mashed, 4 tablespoons (1 ounce) shredded reduced-fat Cheddar cheese (such as Kraft 2% Milk Sharp Cheddar or Cabot Light Vermont Cheddar 50%), and 3 tablespoons salsa. Roll and serve. Have 1 cup baby carrots. Add an apple for dessert.

23. Spinach Bleu Cheese Salad**

Toss together 2 cups spinach (save time by buying pre-washed bagged spinach) and 1 small tomato cut in wedges or 6 cherry tomatoes. Top with 2 tablespoons crumbled Bleu cheese; 2 hard-boiled eggs, sliced; and 1½ table-spoons reduced-fat salad dressing of your choice. Serve with 2 slices rye crisp bread slices (such as Wasa).

24. Stuffed Pockets and Soup

Microwave according to package directions either Lean Pockets (Turkey, Broccoli, and Cheese or Chicken Broc-coli Supreme) or Amy's (Vegetarian Pizza in a Pocket, Broccoli and Cheese in a Pocket, or Soy Cheese Veggie Pizza in a Pocket), or similar frozen pocket (check label for 250–280 calories, 7–10 grams fat). Serve with 1 cup lentil soup (canned is fine) heated with 1 cup fresh spinach (get prewashed, bagged spinach for convenience).

25. Grilled Cheese and Tomato Sandwich**

Between 2 slices whole wheat bread place 2 ounces (usu-ally 2 slices) of reduced-fat cheese (check label for no more than 5 grams fat per slice, as in Borden's 2% Amer-ican cheese singles or Cabot Light Vermont Cheddar 50% Singles) and 3 slices tomato. Grill on a nonstick fry-ing pan sprayed with Pam or in the toaster oven until melted. Serve with 1 cup raw vegetables of your choice—such as cherry tomatoes, green or red pepper slices, or baby carrots—and 10 reduced-fat tortilla chips.

26. Black Bean Soup with Sour Cream

To 1½ cups black bean soup (canned soup is fine) add 1 cup fresh spinach (save time by buying it prewashed and bagged); heat until spinach wilts down. Top with 2 table-spoons reduced-fat sour cream. Serve with ½ cup baby carrots, 8 Reduced Fat Triscuits (or 130 calories' worth of another whole grain cracker), and ½ ounce reduced-fat Cheddar cheese.

27. Pita Vegetable Pizza**
Slice a 6½-inch whole wheat pita (about 170 calories) lengthwise to produce 2 rounds. Spread each round with 1½ tablespoons pizza sauce or thick spaghetti sauce, ¼ cup chopped mushrooms, zucchini, peppers, or other vegetables; and 4 tablespoons (1 ounce) shredded part-skim mozzarella. Heat in oven or toaster oven at 350°F for 8 minutes or until mozzarella just melts. Serve with ½ cup celery sticks. Have an orange for dessert.

28. Baked Potato, Broccoli, and Cheese
Top 1 baked potato (2⅓ inches in diameter and 4¾ inches long) with 6 tablespoons (1½ ounces) shredded, reduced-fat Cheddar cheese (such as Kraft 2% Milk Sharp Cheddar or Cabot Light Vermont Cheddar 50%), and 1 cup cooked chopped broccoli (frozen, microwaved broccoli is fine). Have a small apple for dessert.

29. Smoked Turkey and Cranberry Sandwich***
Spread 2 slices whole wheat bread each with ½ table-spoon reduced-fat mayonnaise. Fill with 2 slices (2 ounces) smoked turkey sliced for sandwiches (check la-bel for no more than 2 grams fat per ounce), 2 table-spoons cranberry sauce, and a piece of romaine lettuce. Serve with 1 cup sliced celery sticks. Have an apple for dessert.

30. Turkey/Avocado/Bacon Wrap***
On an 8- or 9-inch tortilla (preferably whole wheat), place 3 slices (3 ounces) turkey breast sliced for sand-wiches (check label for no more than 2 grams fat per slice), 1 strip bacon, crumbled (save time by microwav-

ing precooked bacon like Oscar Mayer Ready-to-Serve Bacon), 2 tablespoons diced avocado, and 2 slices tomato (optional: 1 tablespoon salsa). Roll and serve with ½ cup baby carrots and 5 baked tortilla chips.

AFTERNOON SNACK CHOICES

Some of these menu options are as simple as grabbing an apple and a half-pint of milk. Others require a little more planning. All are great for nourishing your body and for staving off midafternoon binges. The average snack delivers about 215 calories, 3 grams of total fat, 1 gram of saturated fat, 35 grams of carbohydrates, 10 grams of protein, 10 milligrams of cholesterol, 194 milligrams of sodium, 3 grams of fiber, and 245 milligrams of calcium.

You'll notice that the menu options are divided into three categories. You can choose one Double Snack, which combines a high-calcium food with a fruit, or you can pair a Calcium Snack with a Fruit Snack. Either way, you'll be getting a healthy mix of nutrients. If you're having yogurt, remember to look for a nonfat variety that has about 120 calories per cup, like Dannon Light 'n Fit.

If you prefer to design your own snack, make sure it meets these basic nutrition guidelines.

- Aim for no more than 215 calories.
- Include two servings of fruit (one serving equals ½ cup cut-up fruit or berries, one small piece of fruit, or ¾ cup citrus juice).
- Also include 1 cup of milk, yogurt, or calcium-fortified soy milk, or 1 ounce of reduced-fat cheese.

Calcium Snacks
If you pick an item from this list, you can pair it with one of the Fruit Snacks.

1. Classic Refresher

Drink 1 cup (a half-pint carton) of chilled nonfat milk.
Serve with 1½ graham crackers (one graham cracker is
about 5 inches by 2½ inches) or other crackers totaling
90 calories.

2. Vegetarian Refresher

Drink 1 cup or an 8–9 ounce box of chilled vanilla or
other flavored, low-fat, calcium-fortified soy milk (for
convenience, get Edensoy Extra Original 8.45-ounce cartons) with 1 graham cracker (about 5 inches by 2½ inches)
or other crackers totaling 60 calories.

3. Yogurt Your Way

Have 1 cup (8 ounces) nonfat yogurt in your choice of
flavors (check label for about 120 calories per cup, as in
Dannon Light 'n Fit) topped with 4 teaspoons trail mix.

4. Maple Milk

Heat 1 cup nonfat milk or low-fat, calcium-fortified
vanilla soy milk; stir in 1 teaspoon maple syrup. Serve
with ½ ounce pretzels (about 5 three-ring pretzels).

5. Almond Milk

Add a few drops almond extract to 1 cup of nonfat milk
or low-fat, calcium-fortified vanilla soy milk, cold or
heated. Serve with 1½ graham crackers (one graham
cracker is about 5 inches by 2½ inches) or other crackers
totaling 90 calories.

6. Café au Lait

Mix together 1 cup hot brewed or instant coffee (regular
or decaf) and 1 cup hot nonfat milk or low-fat, calcium-
fortified vanilla soy milk plus 1 teaspoon of sugar, if desired. Serve with 1 graham cracker (about 5 inches by 2½
inches) or other crackers totaling 60 calories.

7. Iced Café au Lait

Mix together 1 cup cold nonfat milk or low-fat, calcium-fortified plain soy milk with 1 cup room-temperature brewed coffee. Add ice and 1 teaspoon sugar if desired. Serve with 1 graham cracker (about 5 inches by 2½ inches) or other crackers totaling 60 calories.

8. Cheese and a Pickle** ***

Have 2 individually wrapped wedges of spreadable Laughing Cow Light—we like the French Onion and Garlic & Herb varieties—or about 70 calories' worth of other cheese spread on 4 Reduced Fat Triscuits (or 65 calories' worth of another whole grain cracker), with a pickle of your choice.

9. Cheese and a Crunch**

Have 1½ slices (1½ ounces) reduced-fat American cheese (less than 5 grams fat per ounce, such as Borden's 2% American cheese singles) wrapped around a stick of celery. (Optional: Dip in hot and spicy mustard.) Serve with 4 Reduced Fat Triscuits (or 65 calories' worth of another whole grain cracker).

10. Hot Chocolate

Heat 1 cup nonfat milk. Add ½ tablespoon chocolate syrup such as Hershey's. (Optional: Add a few drops vanilla extract and top with 2 tablespoons canned whipped cream.) Serve with 1 graham cracker (about 5 inches by 2½ inches) or other crackers totaling 60 calories.

11. Chocolate Milk

Mix 1 cup cold nonfat milk or low-fat, calcium-fortified plain or vanilla soy milk with ½ tablespoon chocolate syrup such as Hershey's. Serve with ½ ounce pretzels (about 5 three-ring pretzels).

12. Strawberry Milk

Mix 1 cup cold nonfat milk or low-fat, calcium-fortified plain or vanilla soy milk with 2 teaspoons strawberry powder such as Nesquik. Serve with 1 graham cracker (about 5 inches by 2½ inches) or other crackers totaling 60 calories.

Fruit Snacks

The items in this list go with the Calcium Snacks; choose one of each for a nutritionally balanced nosh.

13. Just Fruit

Have 1 apple, pear, orange, peach, small banana, or other piece of fruit of your choice.

14. Just Berries

Have ½ to 1 cup berries, such as strawberries, raspberries, blueberries, fresh or frozen (unsweetened).

15. Fruit to Go

Have ½ cup (a 4-ounce container) of fruit canned in its own juice (not syrup). Check labels for around 60 calories per serving. For convenience, use single-serving, peel-top containers, such as Del Monte Fruit Naturals Sliced Peaches in Pear and Peach Juice or Dole Pineapple FruitBowls.

16. Frozen Grapes

Put a cluster of grapes about the size of your fist (½ cup) in the freezer for several hours. Enjoy.

17. Just for You, Baby

Tuck into a jar of baby-food peaches or other baby-food fruit (check label for no more than 70 calories per serving).

18. Apricot Indulgence

Have 3 dried apricots (or 6 halves). As rich and sweet as candy!

19. Ready Raisins
Grab a pack of Sun-Maid's handy ½-ounce minipacks of raisins. A 2-tablespoon serving of raisins is already measured for you.

20. Applesauce Comfort
Applesauce makes a great snack because it feels like comfort food. Try convenient single-serving, peel-top containers with ½ cup applesauce (such as Mott's Natural Style Apple Sauce or Mott's Healthy Harvest—any flavor).

21. Tangy Thirst Quencher
Drink a 6-ounce can of grapefruit juice.

22. Luscious Dried Plums
Enjoy 3 succulent dried plums—that's the sexy new name for prunes! We like the Sunsweet orange essence flavored ones.

23. Portable Fruit Cocktail
Have ½ cup (4 ounces) fruit cocktail canned in juice (no syrup). For convenience, use the single-serving, peel-top containers, such as Del Monte Fruit Naturals Chunky Mixed Fruits in Fruit Juices.

24. Make It Melon
You can have ¼ of a medium cantaloupe, ⅛ of a medium honeydew, or 1 cup of watermelon, cantaloupe, or honeydew pieces.

Double Snacks
Each of the following items combines a fruit with a calcium-rich food for a complete snack. I recommend doing your snacking in the afternoon, to tide you over until dinnertime.

25. Peach Slush
In a blender, combine 1 cup (8 ounces) peach-flavored nonfat yogurt (check label for about 120 calories per cup) with a peeled and sliced, ripe peach or ½ cup canned peach (in juice, not syrup). Add 1 or 2 ice cubes and blend until smooth. Serve with 1 graham cracker (about 5 inches by 2½ inches) or other crackers totaling 60 calories. (For variety, make slush with berry-flavored yogurt and fresh or frozen, unsweetened berries.)

26. Strawberry Soy Milk Smoothie
In a blender, combine until smooth 1 cup low-fat, calcium-fortified vanilla soy milk, half of a ripe banana, and ¼ cup strawberries (fresh or frozen, unsweetened). Serve with 1 graham cracker (about 5 inches by 2½ inches) or other crackers totaling 60 calories. (Alternative: Use 1 cup non-fat milk.)

27. Fruit and Cheese**
Slice a ripe pear or apple; eat with 1 ounce room-temperature reduced-fat Cheddar cheese. Pick a brand like Cabot Light Vermont Cheddar 50%, with about 5 grams fat per ounce; the lower-fat brands don't cut it with fruit. Serve with 4 Reduced Fat Triscuits (or 65 calories' worth of another whole grain cracker).

28. Fruit Blast Yogurt
Mix ½ cup fresh or frozen, unsweetened blueberries or strawberries or any chopped fruit with 1 cup (8 ounces) nonfat berry-flavored yogurt (check label for about 120 calories per cup). Sprinkle with 2 tablespoons low-fat granola.

29. Banana Smoothie
In a blender, combine until smooth: ½ cup nonfat milk, half of a ripe banana, and ½ cup (4 ounces) nonfat vanilla yogurt (check label for about 120 calories per cup). Blend in 1 or 2 ice cubes and a few drops vanilla extract. Serve with ½ ounce pretzels (about 5 three-ring pretzels).

30. Tropical Yogurt

Stir 2 tablespoons tropical dried fruit mix into 1 cup (8 ounces) nonfat pineapple- or apricot-flavored yogurt (check label for about 120 calories per cup). Stir in a few drops coconut extract. Serve with 1 graham cracker (about 5 inches by 2½ inches) or other crackers totaling 60 calories.

DINNER CHOICES

What's for dinner? Take your pick! Every one of these menu options is convenient, delicious, and oh-so-nutritious. The average meal provides 515 calories, 13 grams of total fat, 4 grams of saturated fat, 70 grams of carbohydrates, 30 grams of protein, 86 milligrams of cholesterol, 990 milligrams of sodium, 8 grams of fiber, and 240 milligrams of calcium.

If you enjoy dabbling in the kitchen, feel free to design your own dinner. The criteria couldn't be simpler:

- No more than 515 calories
- Two servings of vegetables (one serving equals 1 cup of raw leafy greens; ½ cup of other vegetables, cooked or raw; or ¾ cup of tomato or vegetable juice)

Effortless Home Cooking

As long as you can open a can or operate a microwave, all these delicious meals can be yours in minutes.

1. Lentil Soup and French Bread***

Heat 2 cups lentil soup (such as approximately one 19-ounce can of Progresso Classics Lentil Soup). Serve with a large slice (about 6 inches long) of warm French bread (for example, ⅙ of Pillsbury's Crusty French Loaf, in refrigerated cans) spread with 2 teaspoons butter or trans-free margarine and 1 cup of red pepper strips. Have an apple for dessert.

2. Pizza and Beer!** ***

Have 1 slice of a large (14-inch) pizza or 1½ slices of a medium (12-inch) pizza topped with two vegetables, such as mushrooms and green pepper. Use only medium- or thin-crust pizza (such as Domino's Hand-Tossed Pizza). For frozen pizza, check labels, and have 265–280 calories' worth. Serve with a salad: 1 cup mixed greens, ½ cup chopped vegetable of your choice, such as tomato, pepper, carrot, etc., with 1½ tablespoons reduced-calorie dressing. Have a 12-ounce can of light beer.

3. Chicken and Veggies

Microwave according to package directions Lean Cuisine Hearty Portions Chicken Florentine or Uncle Ben's Rice Bowl Teriyaki Chicken, or similar frozen meal (check labels for about 370–380 calories, 4–9 grams fat). Serve with 1 cup raw veggies (such as red pepper strips and cucumber sticks) or 1 cup cooked veggies (such as steamed or microwaved broccoli). Have a cup of grapes for dessert.

4. Breakfast for Dinner

Make 2 eggs your way: poached, soft-boiled, or scrambled in a nonstick pan sprayed with butter-flavored Pam. Serve with 2 slices whole wheat toast spread with 1 teaspoon diet margarine (such as Smart Beat Super Light or I Can't Believe It's Not Butter Light) and 2 teaspoons of jam or jelly on each. Have a 6-ounce glass of orange juice.

5. Tortellini, Manicotti, and Lasagna** ***

Microwave according to package directions Healthy Choice Bowls Cheese Tortellini; Healthy Choice Manicotti with Three Cheeses; Amy's Tofu Vegetable Lasagna; or similar frozen food (check label for 300–330 calories, 9–12 grams fat). Add a salad made of 1 cup romaine lettuce or mixed greens, ½ cup chopped vegetables of your choice (such as tomato or cucumber) tossed with 2 tablespoons reduced-calorie salad dressing. Have a pear (or 1 cup pear canned in juice) for dessert.

6. Veggie Burger on the Ranch***

Microwave or grill a vegetable burger according to package directions. Choose patties in the 110–130 calorie range (like The Original Gardenburger or Amy's California Veggie Burger). Place on a whole grain bun spread with 1–2 tablespoons reduced-calorie ranch (or Caesar) dressing. (Optional: Instead of dressing, use mustard and ketchup to taste.) Add 2 thick slices tomato and 2 slices romaine lettuce. Serve with a ½ cup of raw veggies (like carrot and celery sticks) and ⅓ cup baked beans. Enjoy a 12-ounce light beer with dinner.

7. Amy's Skillet Meal Pasta and Vegetables Alfredo**
Serves 2

Add contents of package along with 1 cup chopped broccoli (fresh or frozen) to a nonstick skillet sprayed with Pam. Cook according to package directions. At the last minute, stir in ½ cup cooked skinless chicken strips (such as Perdue Short Cuts or Louis Rich Carving Board). Eat half for one serving. Have a 6-ounce glass of wine or a 12-ounce can of light beer.

8. Cereal for Dinner

In a big bowl, put 180 calories' worth of your favorite cereal (that's a scant cup of raisin bran; 1⅔ cup Cheerios; 1⅛ cup Wheat and Corn Chex or Post Shredded Wheat 'N Bran; or for other cereals check labels to figure out what 180 calories translates to in cups). Add 2 tablespoons sunflower or pumpkin seeds; 1 cup fresh or frozen, unsweetened blueberries or fruit of your choice; and top with 1 cup nonfat milk. Serve with ¾ cup of orange juice.

9. Beef and Veggies

Microwave according to package directions Lean Cuisine Café Classics Teriyaki Steak or similar frozen meal (check label for 370–380 calories, 4–9 grams fat). Add a salad: 1 cup romaine lettuce or mixed greens (save time

with prewashed, bagged greens) and ½ cup cherry tomatoes or other vegetable of your choice. Dress with 1 tablespoon reduced-calorie dressing. Have an orange for
dessert.

10. Soup and Grilled Cheese** ***

Heat 1½ cups minestrone soup (such as Progresso Classics Minestrone or any other that's around 125 calories
per cup). Grilled cheese sandwich: Spread 2 slices whole
wheat bread with 1 teaspoon diet margarine (such as
Smart Beat Super Light or I Can't Believe It's Not Butter
Light) each. With buttered sides out, place 2 slices (2
ounces) reduced-fat cheese (no more than 5 grams of fat
per ounce, such as Borden's 2% American cheese singles
or Cabot Light Cheddar 50% Singles) and 3 slices tomato
between bread slices. Grill in nonstick pan sprayed with
Pam or in toaster oven until cheese melts.

11. Vegetarian Chili with Cornbread***

Heat 1 cup canned vegetarian chili. Serve with a 2-inch
by 4-inch piece of cornbread (about 2 ounces; check your
supermarket bakery department) and a heaping cup of
carrot and celery sticks.

12. Fettuccine Alfredo

Microwave according to package directions Lean Cuisine
Hearty Portions Chicken Fettucine with Broccoli, or similar frozen meal (check label for 400–415 calories, 9–15
grams fat). Steam or microwave ½ cup fresh or frozen
broccoli. Transfer to plate. Pour chicken fettuccine over
broccoli. Serve with a 4-ounce glass of wine.

13. Seafood Dinner

Microwave according to package directions Lean Cuisine
Baked Fish, Healthy Choice Lemon Pepper Fish, or similar frozen meal (check label for 290–320 calories, 6–8 g
fat). Add 1 cup steamed or microwaved vegetables, fresh
or frozen, tossed with a spritz of lemon juice and 1 tea-

spoon olive oil. Serve with a 1-ounce dinner roll (about the size of a tennis ball).

Only a *Little* Cooking Required

Since these menu options serve two, you can make dinner for yourself and your partner. You'll reap tons of brownie points!

14. *Waffles Florentine*** ***
Serves 2 (2 waffles each)

Toast 4 whole grain frozen waffles (check label for about 180 calories for 2 waffles) and microwave a 9-ounce microwavable bag of fresh baby spinach such as Ready Pac brand (or 2 cups frozen chopped spinach) according to package directions (about 3 minutes). Fry 4 eggs in a nonstick skillet sprayed with Pam. Top each waffle with 1 egg and ¼ of the spinach (about ½ cup) and 1 tablespoon of grated Parmesan cheese. Serve with an 8-ounce glass of orange juice.

15. *Southwestern Beans, Rice, and Cheese****
Serves 2

Microwave one Cascadian Farm Aztec Organic Vegetarian Meal (a frozen medley of black beans, brown rice, corn, red peppers, wheat berries, garlic, and spices) according to package directions; set aside, covered. Microwave a microwave-ready 9-ounce bag of fresh baby spinach such as Ready Pac brand (or 2 cups frozen chopped spinach) according to package directions (about 3 minutes). Add cooked spinach to beans and rice. Divide mixture between 2 plates; add a heaping ⅓ cup (2 ounces) cooked chicken strips (Perdue Short Cuts or Louis Rich Carving Board)—for a woman's portion, omit chicken strips. Top each plate with 4 tablespoons Parmesan cheese and microwave for 1 minute to melt cheese. Have 1½ cups canteloupe cubes for dessert.

16. Chicken Cacciatore and Wine***
Serves 2

In a medium (12-inch) heavy-bottomed skillet, place 2 skinless chicken thighs or half-breasts. Cover with 2 cups of your favorite chunky tomato-based meatless spaghetti sauce (sauce with mushrooms works well here). Simmer, covered, for 30 minutes or until chicken is cooked all the way through. Meanwhile boil 1 cup dry penne or other short, tubular pasta (becomes approximately 2 cups cooked). In each bowl place ¾ cup cooked pasta topped with 1 thigh or breast and half the tomato sauce. Serve with a 6-ounce glass of wine. (Women following the Ice Cream Diet should omit half the chicken and have a 3-ounce glass of wine.)

17. Elegant Salmon, Couscous, and Asparagus
Serves 2

In a small, 1½-quart baking dish, pour 1 cup white wine and 1 cup water. Add 5 peppercorns, a whole clove, 2 bay leaves, and a peeled clove of garlic. Put in oven at 350°F. When it comes to a simmer, add two 3-ounce pieces of boneless salmon fillet. Cook skin-side down for 8 minutes or until just done all the way through. With a slotted spoon, remove salmon from liquid. Serve each piece of salmon with 1 cup whole wheat couscous (made according to package directions starting with ½ cup dry couscous for 2 servings, as in Fantastic brand) and 1 cup steamed or microwaved asparagus with a spritz of lemon. Add a 4-ounce glass of wine.

18. Broccoli Pasta with Shrimp
Serves 2

In a medium pot, cook according to package directions 1⅓ cups dry whole wheat pasta (ziti, penne, or other short pasta). While pasta is cooking, in a large nonstick skillet over medium heat, add 1 tablespoon olive oil or canola oil and a clove of minced garlic (or 1 teaspoon garlic powder). Sauté garlic for 30 seconds, then add 15 large or 24 medium shrimp (5 ounces), either fresh or frozen and thawed. Cook until shrimp turn pink, about 4–5 minutes, stirring constantly. Remove shrimp and garlic, add 1 teaspoon olive oil, and sauté 1½ cups chopped fresh or frozen chopped broccoli until tender. Drain pasta when done. Mix with broccoli. Serve half of the broccoli-pasta mixture with half of the shrimp. Start the meal with a 6-ounce glass of V8, and accompany meal with 4-ounce glass of wine.

19. Four-Minute Parmesan Spinach with Salmon**
Serves 2

Microwave a microwave-ready 9-ounce bag of fresh spinach such as Ready Pac brand (or 2 cups frozen chopped spinach) according to package directions (about 3 minutes). Carefully remove hot spinach from bag and fork out 1 cup spinach in each of 2 microwave-safe bowls. In each bowl add a heaping ⅓ cup cooked salmon from uneaten portion you brought home from a restaurant meal such as #30 (alternative: use ⅓ cup cooked chicken strips like Perdue Short Cuts or Louis Rich Carving Board). Sprinkle each bowl with 3 tablespoons Parmesan cheese and microwave about 30–45 seconds, or until cheese begins to melt. Serve with 2 slices whole wheat bread and a 4-ounce glass of wine.

Eating Out

Now we'll show you how to take your diet out for dinner. Order any of these favorite menu items, and you'll still have calories to spare for your ice cream nightcap!

20. Boston Market Chicken Dinner** ***

Order a Quarter Dark Meat Chicken (ask for no skin) or a Quarter White Meat Chicken (ask for no skin or wing). Have a side of Mashed Potatoes (¾ cup). Add a side of Steamed Vegetable Medley or Herbed Sweet Corn (ask for a heaping serving, about a cup). Have half the Cornbread that comes with your meal.

21. Spaghetti with Red Sauce and Seafood
At Olive Garden, order Shrimp Primavera; have half, take the rest home. In other restaurants, 1¼ cup spaghetti with about ½-cup tomato sauce and 2½ ounces seafood—about 14 large shrimp, 9 mussels, or 8 clams. At Olive Garden or elsewhere, add a side salad (1 cup mixed greens); order reduced-calorie dressing on the side and use 1 tablespoon. Enjoy a small (4-ounce) glass of wine.

22. Olive Garden Chicken Giardino
This dish features vegetables and chicken tossed with pasta in a lemon-herb sauce. Have the entire dinner entrée, including side salad, with 4 ounces red wine.

23. A Taste of Greece or the Middle East
Order chicken and vegetable kabob. Have all the skewered vegetables and about 3 ounces chicken (usually about half the total chicken). Take leftover chicken home. Have a side Greek salad (at least 1 cup greens; 2 tablespoons feta; order dressing on the side and use 1 tablespoon.) Eat 1¼ cups rice.

24. A Taste of China***
Order beef and broccoli; chicken and broccoli; or shrimp and broccoli. Or these same dishes with mixed vegetables instead of broccoli. Your strategy: Ask for more vegetables than beef, chicken, or shrimp, and ask them to stir-fry in very little oil. Have 1½ cup entrée with 1 cup steamed rice. If they won't accommodate your requests for less oil, more veggies, etc., then cut back to 1¼ cup entrée with 1 cup steamed rice.

25. Dinner at the Mall***
At Au Bon Pain order a medium serving (12 ounces) of Southwest Vegetable Soup and a Fields 'n Feta Wrap. Eat only half the wrap—these are huge!—and take the rest home.

26. Another Dinner at the Mall** ***
At Schlotzsky's Deli have any of the following sand-wiches in the small size: Santa Fe Chicken, Chicken Club, or Corned Beef. Order a small Garden Salad; use no more than ⅓ packet Light Italian dressing (1 table-spoon).

27. A Stop at Wendy's** ***
Have the large-size chili topped with 2 tablespoons Cheddar cheese, accompanied with 3 packs Saltines (6 crackers). Order the side salad; use ⅓ of a packet of reduced-fat dressing.

28. Quarter Pounder**
Order a ¼-pound burger at Wendy's or McDonald's with-out mayonnaise (ketchup and mustard are fine). When you get home, drink a 6-ounce can of V8. Have an apple for dessert.

29. Mac and Cheese at the Diner** ***
Start with chicken noodle soup—eat about 1½ cups. Or-der mac and cheese (have 1 cup) with 2 side vegetables (such as green beans and carrots). Try them all served on the same plate so you can mix them up in a cheesy pasta medley.

30. Grilled Salmon
At TGI Friday's, order the Jack Daniel's Salmon (tell your waiter not to bring extra sauce). Have a piece of salmon the size of a deck of cards (take the rest home—use it in #19 in this section). This comes with chef's veg-etables; request that they be steamed or cooked in minimal oil. Also, ask for your baked potato plain, and add 1 pat butter. Use the same strategy when ordering salmon in other restaurants. ·

PART IV

Special Treats

CHAPTER ELEVEN

When You Must Splurge

I hope you've had a chance to do some taste testing of your own, so you're convinced—as I am—that lower-calorie ice creams can be just as smooth and flavorful as their premium counterparts. The beauty of the low-cal varieties—those that deliver no more than 125 calories per ½-cup serving—is that you can enjoy a nice-size portion every day without blowing your calorie budget. In other words, you can eat ice cream *and* lose weight!

But perhaps you're the sort of person who is convinced that the words "low-calorie" and "ice cream" shouldn't even be uttered in the same sentence. As an ice cream purist, you have a lot in common with members of a national organization called the Ice Screamers. These people are besotted with their butter pecan, passionate about their pistachio, rhapsodic about their fudge ripple. Low-calorie ice cream? Perish the thought! As one Ice Screamer proclaimed on the organization's Web site (www.icescreamers.com), "Really good ice cream is cream and sugar and calories and fat!"

To accommodate the occasional days when the Ice Screamer in you simply *demands* a taste of high-calorie ice cream—from Breyer's Chocolate Mint at 170 calories per ½-cup serving to Häagen-Dazs Chocolate Peanut Butter at 360 calories per ½-cup serving—we've created a Splurge

Formula. Following the formula, you'll be able to enjoy the most extravagantly super-premium ice cream and still stay within a calorie limit that supports weight loss (that's 1,500 calories per day for women, 2,000 calories per day for men).

As you'll soon see, on the days you indulge in a high-cal ice cream, you'll be exceeding what's considered a healthy cutoff for saturated fat, even though you're on target with your calories. Eating too much saturated fat will raise your cholesterol and threaten your heart. So the registered dietitian in me wants to make clear up front: *The Splurge Formula is not for everyday use.* Out of respect for your heart and your long-term good health, *please* limit your splurges to no more than once every 2 weeks. And once you've had your splurge, get right back on the regular Ice Cream Diet eating plan. That way, you continue to lose weight while getting the optimum nutrition your body needs.

Happily, thanks to the super-healthy Ice Cream Diet mix-and-match menus, a high-fat splurge now and then won't do any harm. You can relax and let yourself enjoy every spoonful! So as promised, here's our Splurge Formula—the secret that keeps high-cal Rocky Road from turning into Lumpy Hips on *you*.

DOING THE NUMBERS

With the Splurge Formula, you can choose *any* ice cream you desire. You just need to figure out how much you can have based on a 250-calorie limit if you're a woman and a 375-calorie limit if you're a man. These are the ice cream calorie allowances that make the Ice Cream Diet work. The advantage: By doing this, you can eat *any* ice cream and continue to lose weight. The disadvantage: If you go with a high-cal variety, you'll be getting less than your usual serving (1 cup for women, 1½ cups for men)—in some cases, a lot less.

If the thought of eating just a little ice cream is just too depressing, you may want to stick with lower-calorie varieties so you can indulge in larger portions. But if you're intrigued by the idea of enjoying even a taste of your favorite super-premium now and then, get out your calculator and do the following math. You'll end up with a serving size that fits the Ice Cream Diet perfectly.

1. On the Nutrition Facts label, find the number of calories per ½-cup serving.
2. If you're a woman, divide 2,000 by the number of calories per serving. This tells you the exact number of tablespoons that supplies 250 calories' worth of ice cream. If you're a man, divide 3,000 by the number of calories per serving to get the number of tablespoons that contains 375 calories' worth of ice cream.
3. Convert tablespoons into cups using "Conversions for the Splurge Formula" on the next page. Now you know the serving size for your splurge.

Let's test the formula by running through an example together. Suppose a certain guy just loves Ben & Jerry's Pistachio Pistachio. Here's what he has to do.

1. Find the number of calories per ½-cup serving. *Answer: 250 calories*.
2. Divide 3,000 by 250. *Answer: 12.* This means 12 tablespoons of Ben & Jerry's Pistachio Pistachio has 375 calories, a man's ice cream calorie allowance on the Ice Cream Diet.
3. Convert 12 tablespoons into cups. *Answer: ¾ cup.* So our guy can have ¾ cup of Ben & Jerry's Pistachio Pistachio ice cream, plus a day's worth of Ice Cream Diet meals and snacks, and stay on track for weight loss.

So why can't you do this every day—have a smaller portion of a higher-calorie ice cream, as long as you don't mind the skimpy servings? Because of all that saturated fat lurking in almost all higher-cal ice creams. You'll be getting gobs of it, even if you stay within your calorie budget. For example, that ¾ cup of Ben & Jerry's Pistachio Pistachio—even though it doesn't exceed a man's 375-calorie ice cream al-

---

CONVERSIONS FOR THE SPLURGE FORMULA

Use this chart to help figure out the serving size for your splurge. Remember, a ½-cup serving of ice cream is about the size of a tennis ball.

2 tablespoons = ⅛ cup
4 tablespoons = ¼ cup
6 tablespoons = ⅜ cup
8 tablespoons = ½ cup
10 tablespoons = ⅝ cup
12 tablespoons = ¾ cup
14 tablespoons = ⅞ cup
16 tablespoons = 1 cup

---

lowance—actually delivers 15 grams of saturated fat. That's all a guy should have in *1 whole day*.

Using the Splurge Formula, a woman could have ½ cup of Ben & Jerry's Pistachio Pistachio and stick with her 250-calorie ice cream allowance. But that ½ cup contains 10 grams of saturated fat, just 1 gram shy of a woman's daily saturated fat limit.

This is why I recommend that you use the Splurge Formula no more than once every 2 weeks. Because we've designed the meals on the Ice Cream Diet to be very low in saturated fat, a biweekly splurge should be okay. So relax and enjoy!

SERVING SIZE MATTERS

Happily, a few higher-calorie frozen desserts come *without* all that saturated fat. One example is Ben & Jerry's Low-Fat Cherry Garcia Frozen Yogurt. Each ½-cup serving contains 170 calories, but only 2 grams of saturated fat. Following the Splurge Formula, a woman could have ¾ cup of ice cream for 250 calories and a relatively modest 3 grams of saturated fat. For a man, 1⅛ cups would supply 375 calories and a little over 4 grams of saturated fat. If you can be satisfied with the smaller servings, you're welcome to enjoy products like

Ben & Jerry's Low-Fat Cherry Garcia Frozen Yogurt—
higher in calories but low in fat—every day you're on the Ice
Cream Diet.

The question is: Can you *really* be satisfied with the
smaller servings? If you can, go for it! But please, please
don't fudge it. Believe me, I know from firsthand experience
how easily "portion creep" can overrun the very best inten-
tions to stick with appropriate serving sizes. As portions get
bigger, your progress toward your weight-loss goal will diminish, along with the improved health and quality of life
you've been enjoying as a result. If you're concerned that
might happen, I say, Why even go there? Stick with the
wonderful low-calorie ice creams that you've already discovered.

In fact, you can turn your low-cal favorites into a some-
time splurge by dressing them up as sundaes. If you're a
woman, start with an ice cream that contains 125 calories or
less per ½-cup serving. Because your total ice cream allowance is 250 calories, you can have ½ cup of ice cream
and put the remaining 125 calories toward toppings. (For
topping suggestions and their calorie counts per serving, see
"Dressing Up Vanilla" on page 148.) If you're a guy, you can
dish out a full cup of ice cream—250 calories' worth—and
have 125 calories left over for toppings. You'll stay within
your 375-calorie ice cream allowance.

For even more variety, turn to chapter 13, "Ice Cream
Dreams and More!" There you'll find 19 easy recipes for
treats like Raspberry Ricotta Swirl, Chocolate Mocha
Frappe, and Icy Mango Shiver. Women can substitute almost
any of these irresistible recipes for their daily cup of ice
cream and not blow their calorie budgets. Men can substitute
any recipe at all! Every one delivers a healthy dose of calcium to boot.

THE UH-OH SPLURGE

Realistically, you will have splurges that you probably
haven't planned for—like when you polish off a pint or

DRESSING UP VANILLA

Start with vanilla, or any flavor, and add "the works" to create your own masterpiece. Here's how various toppings add up, calorie-wise.

TOPPING	SERVING SIZE	CALORIES
Chocolate syrup	2 Tbsp	100
Chocolate syrup, "lite"	2 Tbsp	50
Hot fudge topping	2 Tbsp	130
Hot fudge topping, fat-free	2 Tbsp	100
Butterscotch topping	2 Tbsp	130
Butterscotch topping, fat-free	2 Tbsp	100
Caramel topping	2 Tbsp	120
Caramel topping, fat-free	2 Tbsp	100
Peanut butter, melted	2 Tbsp	190
Whipped cream	1/4 cup	40
Peanuts	2 Tbsp	105
Crème de menthe liqueur	2 Tbsp	62
Coffee liqueur	2 Tbsp	54
Frozen orange juice concentrate	2 Tbsp	56
Toasted wheat germ	2 Tbsp	60
Marshmallow creme	2 Tbsp	40
Maraschino cherry	1	10
Chocolate morsels	1 Tbsp	70
Chocolate sprinkles	1 Tbsp	60
Dark chocolate-covered pretzel	1	50
Fresh strawberries	1/4 cup	20
Sliced bananas	1/4 cup	56

more of ice cream in one sitting. Actually, that isn't a splurge. It's a binge. And it deserves your attention. Here's what to do.

Start counting. First, I recommend sitting down and figuring out just how many calories you've eaten, as painful as that might be. With a super-premium ice cream like Häagen-Dazs Chocolate Peanut Butter, you'd be getting 1,440 calories from a whole pint (based on 360 calories per ½ cup). But even Healthy Choice Low Fat Cherry Chocolate Chunk isn't so healthy if you down an entire pint for 440 calories (110 calories per ½ cup). Either way, regardless of whether you're a man or a woman, you've gone way over the ice cream calorie allowance that's built in to the Ice Cream Diet.

Now you may be wondering, What's the point of counting calories after the fact? After all, the damage is done. The point is this: In a binge situation, all of us have a very human tendency to just ignore what we've done. I suspect we subconsciously convince ourselves that if we never actually know how many calories we've eaten, they really don't count.

My experience, with myself and with clients, is that focusing on the exact calorie tab for a binge is at least one way to discourage a repeat performance. Once you realize just what you've done to your body, you may be less inclined to subject it to the same treatment anytime soon.

Adopt a mantra. The next time you're tempted to binge, you'll say to yourself, "No, I'm not going to down that pint of ice cream." But deep down, you might feel deprived, even sorry for yourself. At that moment, I hope you'll invoke the mantra that psychologist Stephen P. Gullo, Ph.D., a New York City weight-loss expert, teaches to his clients: "Saying no to a binge food? *It's not deprivation—it's liberation!*"

By successfully overcoming your desire to binge, you are freeing yourself from the tyranny of too many calories and too many pounds. Try to focus on that rather than any feeling of deprivation. I believe Dr. Gullo's powerful insight can help almost anyone.

Stay the course. Above all else, don't let your weight-loss efforts succumb to negative thinking: "All is lost. I've thrown away the progress I made. Why should I go back to my healthy eating plan?" Instead, acknowledge all the times

BEST AIR YOU'VE EVER HAD!

Of all the foods we eat, ice cream may be one of the most complex—a creamy, ethereal mixture of milk fat, microscopic ice crystals, sugar, milk protein, and air bubbles. To find out how it gets that way, we asked Cary Frye, vice president of regulatory affairs for the International Dairy Foods Association in Washington, D.C., to give us a crash course in making commercial ice cream.

The process begins with milk, cream, and nonfat milk solids in stainless steel vats holding 50 to 3,000 gallons, or sometimes more. The more cream, the higher the fat content of the finished product. Similarly, the more nonfat milk solids, the more calcium.

As the basic ingredients churn inside the vats, sweeteners like corn syrup and cane sugar are added, followed by stabilizers and emulsifiers like guar gum, carrageenan, lecithin, locust bean gum, and even egg yolks. These help produce a creamy texture and keep large ice crystals from forming.

Next, the mixture is pasteurized to kill bacteria and homogenized to break down the milk-fat globules. Then, inside special freezers, stainless steel "dashers" beat in tiny air pockets to prevent the ice cream from becoming a solid, rocklike mass as it freezes. Though not listed on the label, the amount of air, or overrun, in ice cream plays an important role in the fat and calorie load.

Super-premium ice creams have the least air, maybe 30 percent. They're heavier, and highest in fat. (High fat, of course, means high calorie.) Premium ice creams might contain 40 percent air; regular ice creams, 45 percent air.

Ice creams that are the least dense have just under 100 percent overrun, the maximum allowable by law. An ice cream with 100 percent overrun actually is 50 percent air! Products like these tend to be softer and melt quickly. They're lower in calories, too.

After coming out of the freezer, the ice cream moves on to a "hardening room," where it's frozen at temperatures below 0°F. (Soft ice cream—including soft-serve ice cream and frozen custard—doesn't go through the hardening process.) The next step? Distribution to eager ice cream lovers everywhere.

you've made good decisions that kept you faithful to the Ice Cream Diet. Stacking up your successes against one little mistake should help put your binge in perspective. Yes, it's a diversion. But it's not a disaster. Put it behind you and get back on track. Stay with the Ice Cream Diet, choosing your next meal or snack from the mix-and-match menus, just as before. And you'll continue to slim down.

TIME TO TAKE STOCK

What if you find yourself bingeing repeatedly—say, more than once every few months? That's a potentially serious situation, one that requires closer examination.

For one thing, if you are bingeing on ice cream, it may be a sign that you shouldn't follow the Ice Cream Diet under any circumstances. For you, ice cream may be a trigger food. In my experience, when most people eat regular balanced meals and also know they can have a forbidden food like ice cream every day, the need to binge is defused. But if that isn't the case for you, then you need to reconsider whether you should be eating ice cream at all. (You still can use the Ice Cream Diet to lose weight, however. For your nighttime snack, simply switch from ice cream to a non-trigger food with the same number of calories—250 for women, 375 for men.)

Bingeing also may be a sign that now is not a good time for you to be dieting. Any weight-loss program requires emotional energy. If you're under exceptional stress—a new job, a sick child, a conflict with a partner—just maintaining your current weight without gaining may be a more realistic goal. Don't ask yourself to take on more than you can deal with at this moment.

Finally, if you are bingeing and can't seem to stop, you'll see the scale climbing. I urge you, if you can, to seek professional help—whether from a registered dietitian or a psychologist who specializes in problems with overeating. Think this seems too drastic? Then consider the high personal price of weighing too much. According to a new report from the American Cancer Society, obesity and poor nutrition now cause as many cancer deaths as cigarettes! If you're overeating, you're not alone. More than half of all Americans must work on conquering this serious threat to good health.

While you may need extra support right now, I hope that by trying the Ice Cream Diet menus, you'll establish a pattern of eating healthy, satisfying, fuss-free meals. This will help you gain control of your eating habits—not by depriving you, but by liberating you from the tyranny of too much food.

CHAPTER TWELVE

Surviving the Ice Cream Shops

Following the Ice Cream Diet is easy when you're on your home turf. You've got your premeasured scoop or tennis ball, your special dish, and your ice cream with its Nutrition Facts label—all at your fingertips. These reliable tools, together with the Ice Cream Diet's mix-and-match menus, allow you to have your ice cream and lose weight, too!

It's an entirely different story when you're shopping at the mall or driving down the local fast-food strip, and you find yourself face to face with temptation in the guise of an ice cream shop. You could swear you hear your favorite flavor beckoning you to stop by for just a taste, a dish . . . a triple-dip cone!

Relax.

You don't need to keep an ice cream scoop in your back pocket or a tennis ball in your purse to stick with the Ice Cream Diet and stay on track toward your weight-loss goals. Nor do you need to confine your ice cream indulgences to your home.

But if you're thinking of eating ice cream out, you do need to be prepared. That's because at most ice cream specialty stores—from national chains to mom-and-pop shops—you can buy ice creams, frozen yogurts, sundaes, and shakes that will send your calorie count right through the roof and deluge your arteries with saturated fat.

At one national chain, we found a five-scoop banana split that packs 1,290 calories—nearly enough to use up a woman's calorie budget for an entire day! At another, we discovered a regular-size, 16-ounce chocolate shake that delivers 750 calories. And a premium shop's frozen yogurts—which so many people assume are healthier—contain up to 460 calories per 1-cup serving. You get the picture.

Happily, that's only *part* of the picture. In our sleuthing, we also came across some delicious frozen treats that have 125 calories or less per ½-cup serving, which means they're perfect for the Ice Cream Diet. They range from hand-dipped ice creams to soft-serves, including frozen yogurt. You'll find a selection of these blue-ribbon choices in "Top Shop Picks." (For more, refer to the ice cream comparison chart that begins on page 210.) What's the easiest way to do an ice cream shop run without blowing your daily calorie budget? If you can, head for a shop that serves these calorie winners.

Still, you will have occasions when you're faced with a menu board that lists dozens of tempting ice creams and frozen treats—but no calorie information. For those moments, consider this chapter your survival guide.

ONE SIMPLE SECRET

When you're following an eating plan like the Ice Cream Diet, how do you navigate ice cream shops and keep losing weight? We asked two registered dietitians, both spokespersons for the American Dietetic Association, for their advice. What they told us makes things very easy.

Essentially, whenever you venture out for ice cream, you just need to remember one incredibly important rule: "If you want to lose weight," says Edith Hogan, R.D., a Washington, D.C.–based dietitian who counsels private clients, "you must be really serious about watching your serving sizes."

Ideally, you could go on a company's Web site and check

TOP SHOP PICKS

All of the following frozen desserts deliver fewer than 125 calories per $\frac{1}{2}$-cup serving, which means they're just right for the Ice Cream Diet. You can have a full cup if you're a woman, or $1\frac{1}{2}$ cups if you're a man, and stay on track for your weight-loss goal.

All of these products contain calcium, too—though some have less than the optimum levels recommended for the ice creams you eat on a daily basis. That's okay, since your ice cream shop excursions are once-in-a-while treats.

Be aware that products and flavors may change periodically, and even vary from shop to shop within the same chain. We found these when we did our own comparison shopping.

ICE CREAM SHOP	ICE CREAM TYPE	FLAVOR(S)	CALORIES PER $\frac{1}{2}$ CUP OR SMALL PORTION	CALCIUM (% DV)
Baskin Robbins	Soft Serve	Chocolate Banana Twist	100	15
	Nonfat Yogurt	Chocolate Mint	120	15
		Kahlua	110	15
Carvel	No Fat	Vanilla Ice Cream	120	15
TCBY	Soft Serve Nonfat Frozen Yogurt	Golden Vanilla and White Chocolate Mousse	110	10
	No Sugar Added Nonfat Frozen Yogurt	Vanilla, Chocolate, White Chocolate Macadamia Nut, Strawberry	80	10
	Hand-Dipped Lowfat Ice Cream	Raspberry Cheesecake, Banana Pudding, Mint Chocolate Chip, Peanut Butter Fudge Nut	120	10
	Swirl Bar	Orange, Raspberry	80	20

out the serving sizes and calorie counts for its frozen desserts before you patronize one of its shops. Or you could get a nutrition pamphlet right at the shop, if one is available.

But let's assume the worst case: The nutrition information just doesn't exist. "When in doubt," advises Joan Carter, R.D., who teaches nutrition to medical students at Baylor College of Medicine in Houston, "order the smallest serving available."

To make extra-certain you avoid calorie overload when you don't know the calorie count for a hard ice cream, tell the server you want *one* scoop about the size of a tennis ball, which is ½ cup. (If the person can't visualize a tennis ball, suggest using a fist instead. A ½-cup serving is a little smaller than a woman's balled fist, or about half of a man's balled fist.)

The same rule applies for soft-serve ice cream: Ask the server for a squiggle about the size of a tennis ball. If you follow this ½-cup rule, you almost always will stay within the Ice Cream Diet's calorie allowance for your daily ice cream treat—and your weight loss won't be interrupted.

If you don't speak up and explain exactly what you want, you'll probably get twice as much ice cream as you should. According to Hogan, the smallest scoop used in most shops dishes up about 1 cup. Of course, if you get more than you intended, you don't have to eat every bite.

Be prepared to feel a bit shortchanged when you first downsize the quantity of ice cream you order. "We Americans no longer can visualize what 'small' is," Carter says. You may need some time to reset your mental image of how much food you need. But it's one of the smartest things you can do for your waistline, and for your health in general.

When you do find an ice cream that you know is truly lower calorie—125 calories or less per ½ cup—you can have a serving equal to 2 tennis balls (1 cup) if you're a woman, or 3 tennis balls (1½ cups) if you're a man. That's the same generous portion you'd be getting if you were eating your ice cream at home.

MORE SURVIVAL STRATEGIES

Besides paying attention to serving size, you can keep a cap on calories from ice cream shop indulgences by sticking with classic flavors like vanilla, chocolate, and strawberry. Extras like chocolate chunks, peanut butter cups, cookie dough, and candies make calorie counts soar. "The more you add, the more calories you're going to get," Hogan explains. "Simpler is better." Whenever possible, choose low-fat or nonfat ice cream over regular. And don't make the mistake of assuming that frozen yogurts are automatically low cal. They aren't!

In fact, of all frozen desserts, sherbet usually has one of the lower calorie contents—about 100 to 160 calories per ½-cup serving. It also has less calcium. Back in chapter 7, I recommended choosing ice creams that contain 100 milligrams of calcium, or 10 percent of the Daily Value, per ½-cup serving. But since you're doing the ice cream shop thing only as a special treat, not as a daily ritual, a high calcium level isn't as critical.

You can trim a few more calories from your ice cream by ordering it in a cup rather than a cone. "If you do want a cone, steer clear of those giant waffle cones, which can tag on up to 300 calories," Carter recommends.

And when you eat your ice cream, don't sit down. You can burn a few extra calories by walking around. Even better, when you're in the mood for an ice cream shop run, leave your car in the garage and get there on foot or by bicycle instead!

WHAT'S IN A CONE?

Wonder how many calories that cone contributes to your double dip? Here are the numbers.

1 wafer cone (the mostly-air kind)	24 calories
1 cake cone (the rolled kind)	40 calories
1 waffle cone (the giant kind)	120 calories or more

HAVE IT YOUR WAY

Of course, an ice cream shop just wouldn't be an ice cream shop if it didn't offer an array of tempting treats made with—what else?—ice cream. So let's say you really, really want to have a milk shake. No problem: Just order the smallest size available and ask for fat-free or low-fat ice cream. Request an empty cup, too—the smallest size available. Fill it with about 1 cup of shake (about what you'd get in a small container of yogurt) and make that your serving. It's about 250 calories' worth.

What do you do with the rest of your milk shake? If you're with someone, maybe you can share. That's good for more than just controlling your portion. "The focus no longer is on devouring what's in front of you," Edith Hogan explains. "You're enjoying your treat and socializing, too."

Another option: Try Wendy's junior-size Frosty, a milk shake–like dessert that has 170 calories. On the other hand, if you prefer floats to milk shakes, order one made with diet cola or diet root beer and 2 tennis ball–size scoops of nonfat or low-fat ice cream, Carter suggests. That runs about 250 calories, too.

Or suppose sundaes are your weakness. Ask for a tennis ball–size scoop of nonfat or lowfat ice cream and one spoonful—about a tablespoon or a half-dollar–size serving—of topping, Hogan says. Toppings can be deceiving, though. Even that innocuous strawberry is likely to be more sugary syrup than fruit, Joan Carter says. The calories can add up fairly quickly.

But this might be a surprise: One of the lowest-calorie toppings is whipped cream. Since it's mostly air, a 2-tablespoon dollop—about the size of a Ping-Pong ball—has only 20 calories. The trouble is, you get almost a full cup on most sundaes. All that fluff adds 160 calories and 8 grams of artery-clogging saturated fat to your dream dessert. (To size up the calorie contents of other popular toppings, see "Dressing Up Vanilla" on page 148.)

WHAT ARE "DIPPIN' DOTS"?

Their manufacturer bills them as "The Ice Cream of the Future." But Dippin' Dots are here today—tiny round ice-cream beads, "flash frozen" at supercold temperatures. They're served in cups, and you can eat them with a spoon.

The dots were invented in the late 1980s by Curt Jones, then a research microbiologist in Lexington, Kentucky, who specialized in cryogenics, a method of freezing at extremely low temperatures. Aside from cryogenics, Jones's other passion was ice cream.

Before long, he'd patented his product and opened a shop. Today, Dippin' Dots are sold nationwide at malls, theme parks, and sports arenas.

To try Dippin' Dots on the Ice Cream Diet, order one serving of Nonfat Yogurt (perhaps the Strawberry Cheesecake flavor) for 110 calories; the No-Sugar-Added Vanilla Reduced Fat Ice Cream for 120 calories; Sherbet (maybe the Red Raspberry flavor) for 100 calories; or Fat-Free No-Sugar-Added Fudge for 60 calories. The original Ice Cream Dippin' Dots contain 190 calories and 100 milligrams of calcium per serving. If you order them, eat only ⅔ of your cup. You'll fall below the desired calcium range, but still get to enjoy this unusual treat guilt-free.

You won't find Dippin' Dots at your local supermarket, though. Nor can you store them at home. That's because the dots must be held at −40°F, far colder than your grocer's freezer case or your fridge.

EAT UP AND ENJOY!

Armed with these strategies, you can venture into any ice cream shop with confidence and come out with a treat that satisfies your ice cream tooth but stays within your Ice Cream Diet calorie allowance. In short, you won't derail your weight-loss efforts.

But the experts offer one final piece of advice: Whatever

you order at the ice cream shop, take time to enjoy it. Really savor every cool, creamy spoonful as it slides over your tastebuds.

"Any treat is meant to be enjoyed," Hogan says. "It's all about balance and moderation."

CHAPTER THIRTEEN

Ice Cream Dreams and More!

Even the most ardent of ice cream aficionados might have days when they hanker for something other than their favorite flavors, plain and unadorned. That's why we decided to assemble this collection of recipes: We want you to have choices! You can substitute one of these 19 fabulous treats for your daily serving of ice cream without blowing your calorie budget.

We've provided easy instructions for making your own ice cream sundaes, smoothies, and coolers—plus several luscious desserts that don't contain ice cream or frozen yogurt but do deliver a decent amount of calcium, for those occasions when you really crave a change of pace. None of the recipes exceeds 375 calories per serving, which means guys can take their pick. Women should stick with the ones that supply 250 calories or less per serving—which still offers lots of choices!

All of the recipes are low in fat, and all supply some calcium. Those marked with an asterisk (*) will contribute at least 100 milligrams of calcium, or 10 percent of the Daily Value, to your total daily intake.

TEMPTING DESSERTS

Chocolate Chip Parfait*

If you're a fan of chocolate and coffee, this dessert is bound to become one of your favorites.

2 teaspoons instant espresso powder
1/2 cup boiling water
8 fat-free chocolate chip biscotti, crushed
2 2/3 cups fat-free vanilla frozen yogurt
4 teaspoons grated semisweet chocolate

In a small bowl, dissolve the espresso powder in the water. Set aside to cool.

Divide one-third of the biscotti crumbs among 4 parfait glasses. In each glass, layer 1/3 cup of the frozen yogurt, 1 tablespoon of the espresso, and 1/2 teaspoon of the chocolate. Repeat. Top with the remaining biscotti crumbs. Serve immediately or freeze for up to 1 hour.

Serves 4
Per serving: 186 calories, 1.3 g fat, 2 mg cholesterol, 0.2 g fiber, 100 mg sodium, 140 mg calcium

Granola Berry Parfait

This recipe calls for blueberries and strawberries, but feel free to use other fruits based on availability—and, of course, taste!

2 cups fat-free vanilla yogurt
2 cups low-fat granola
1 cup blueberries
1 cup sliced strawberries
2 kiwifruit, peeled and chopped

Layer half of the yogurt, granola, blueberries, strawberries, and kiwifruit in 4 parfait glasses or bowls. Repeat.

Serves 4
Per serving: 333 calories, 3.6 g fat, 2 mg cholesterol, 5.4 g fiber, 160 mg sodium, 50 mg calcium

Pineapple-Coconut Crisp

Fruit crisps topped with ice cream are the perfect healthy ending to almost any meal.

1¼ cups coarsely chopped low-fat gingersnaps
1 cup quick-cooking oats
⅓ cup + ½ cup light brown sugar
⅓ cup sweetened shredded coconut
2 tablespoons butter or margarine
½ teaspoon ground cinnamon
1 pineapple, cut into 1" cubes, or 1 can (16 ounces) pineapple
    tidbits in juice, drained
6 peaches, cut into 1" cubes
¾ cup orange juice
2 tablespoons dark rum or 1 teaspoon rum extract
1 tablespoon cornstarch
1½ pints fat-free vanilla ice cream

Preheat the oven to 375°F. Lightly coat a medium baking dish with nonstick spray.

In a small bowl, combine the gingersnaps, oats, ⅓ cup of the brown sugar, the coconut, butter or margarine, and cinnamon. Using your hands, combine to form coarse crumbs.

In a medium bowl, combine the pineapple, peaches, orange juice, rum or rum extract, cornstarch, and the remaining ½ cup brown sugar. Stir until the brown sugar and cornstarch are dissolved. Pour into the prepared baking dish. Sprinkle with the gingersnap mixture.

Bake for 35 to 40 minutes, or until golden brown and bubbly. Remove to a rack to cool for 15 minutes. To serve, top each portion with ¼ cup of the ice cream.

Serves 12

Per serving: 231 calories, 5 g fat, 0 mg cholesterol, 3 g fiber, 81 mg sodium, 80 mg calcium

Ricotta Coffee Cream*

Rich in taste yet light in calories, this dessert takes just a couple of minutes in the food processor.

 1 container (15 ounces) fat-free ricotta cheese
 1/2 cup cold very strong coffee or espresso
 1/4 cup sugar
 1 teaspoon ground nutmeg

In a food processor, combine the ricotta, coffee or espresso, sugar, and nutmeg. Process for 2 minutes, stopping once to scrape down the sides of the bowl with a rubber spatula.

Turn into 4 serving dishes or glasses and freeze for 20 minutes. If planning to store for more than 30 minutes before serving, cover and place in the refrigerator.

Serves 4
Per serving: 131 calories, 0.2 g fat, 12 mg cholesterol, 0 g fiber, 62 mg sodium, 564 mg calcium

Peach Melba*

Named after Nellie Melba, a famous 19th-century Australian opera star, this dessert is deservedly famous, too.

 2 ripe peaches, peeled and halved
 1 cup water
 1/4 cup honey
 1 package (10 ounces) frozen raspberries, thawed
 1 tablespoon cornstarch
 1 pint fat-free vanilla frozen yogurt

In a medium saucepan, combine the peaches, water, and honey. Cook over medium heat until the peaches are soft, about 5 minutes. Remove the peaches with a slotted spoon and set aside to cool.

Meanwhile, in a medium saucepan, combine the raspberries and cornstarch, stirring until the cornstarch is dissolved. Cook over medium heat until the mixture thickens, about 3 minutes. Remove from the heat and let cool for 10 minutes.

To serve, place a peach half in a dessert dish and top with a scoop of frozen yogurt and the warm raspberry sauce.

Serves 4

Per serving: 254 calories, 0.2 g fat, 2 mg cholesterol, 3.9 g fiber, 72 mg sodium, 104 mg calcium

Raspberry Ricotta Swirl*

In this recipe, fat-free ricotta provides a lush flavor and a creamy texture that could rival your favorite premium ice cream.

1 container (15 ounces) fat-free ricotta cheese
1/3 cup plus 2 tablespoons sugar
1 tablespoon orange juice
2 cups fresh or frozen raspberries
Mint leaves

In a food processor, combine the ricotta, 1/3 cup of the sugar, and the orange juice. Process for 30 seconds, or until creamy and smooth. Transfer the ricotta mixture to a large bowl and refrigerate.

Rinse and dry the food processor bowl, then add the raspberries and puree them with the remaining 2 tablespoons sugar. Dollop over the ricotta mixture.

Using a small knife, cut the raspberry puree through the ricotta mixture to create swirls. Cover and refrigerate for at least 4 hours. Serve garnished with the mint leaves.

Serves 4

Per serving: 202 calories, 0.4 g fat, 12 mg cholesterol, 2.8 g fiber, 58 mg sodium, 576 mg calcium

Bananas Foster*

This updated version of a classic dessert combines fat-free ice cream with bananas and brown sugar.

    1 tablespoon butter or margarine
    2 tablespoons dark brown sugar
    2 tablespoons apple juice concentrate
    1/4 teaspoon ground cinnamon
    3 bananas, cut in half crosswise and halves quartered
        lengthwise
    2 teaspoons vanilla extract
    3 cups fat-free vanilla ice cream

Melt the butter or margarine in a medium nonstick skillet set over medium heat. Add the brown sugar, apple juice concentrate, and cinnamon. Cook, stirring, until the sugar melts.

Add the bananas. Toss to coat well. Cook for 3 to 5 minutes, or until the bananas are tender.

Remove from the heat. Add the vanilla extract. Swirl to combine. Serve the ice cream topped with the bananas and sauce.

Serves 6

Per serving: 226 calories, 2 g fat, 7 mg cholesterol, 2 g fiber, 68 mg sodium, 110 mg calcium

Chocolate Raspberry Sundae*

A fruity chocolate sauce over raspberry frozen yogurt . . . how could you resist?

    1/4 cup light corn syrup
    1/4 cup water
    3 tablespoons all-fruit raspberry spread
    2 tablespoons unsweetened cocoa powder
    2 teaspoons cornstarch
    1/2 teaspoon vanilla extract
    1 pint fat-free raspberry frozen yogurt

In a small saucepan, combine the corn syrup, water, and raspberry spread.

In a small bowl, stir together the cocoa powder and cornstarch.

Add the cocoa mixture to the saucepan and mix well. Cook over medium-low heat until thickened, about 2 minutes. Remove from the heat and stir in the vanilla.

Serve warm or cold over the frozen yogurt.

Serves 4
Per serving: 203 calories, 0.3 g fat, 2 mg cholesterol, 0.2 g fiber, 88 mg sodium, 149 mg calcium

REFRESHING SMOOTHIES AND COOLERS

Chocolate Mocha Frappe*
This drink will cool you off fast!

½ cup boiling water
2 teaspoons instant espresso powder
2 cups fat-free milk
3 tablespoons fat-free chocolate syrup
1 cup crushed ice

In a measuring cup or bowl, combine the water and espresso powder. Stir to dissolve. Pour into an ice-cube tray. Freeze for 2 hours, or until solid.

In a blender, combine the milk, chocolate syrup, and frozen coffee ice cubes. Blend until smooth. Add the ice and blend again until smooth.

Serves 2
Per serving: 147 calories, 1 g fat, 4 mg cholesterol, 1 g fiber, 159 mg sodium, 310 mg calcium

Caribbean Fruit Frappe

One sip of this delightful drink, and you'll be transported to a seaside cabana.

1 1/2 cups chopped pineapple (use fresh or canned in juice, drained)
1 cup low-fat vanilla ice cream
1 cup sliced or chopped peeled fresh or prepared mango
2 tablespoons lime juice
1/2 teaspoon coconut extract

In a blender or food processor, puree the pineapple, ice cream, mango, lime juice, and coconut extract until smooth. Serve in tall glasses.

Serves 4
Per serving: 115 calories, 1.4 g fat, 3 mg cholesterol, 2.7 g fiber, 27 mg sodium, 54 mg calcium
Note: Look for jars of prepared mango slices in the refrigerator section of the produce department or bags of chopped mango in the freezer section.

Berry Berry Smoothie*

Berries are looking so healthy, many nutrition experts now recommend eating some every day.

1/2 cup frozen unsweetened raspberries, thawed
1/2 cup frozen unsweetened strawberries, thawed
3/4 cup unsweetened pineapple juice
1 cup fat-free vanilla yogurt

In a blender, combine the raspberries, strawberries, and pineapple juice. Add the yogurt. Blend until smooth.

Serves 2
Per serving: 195 calories, 1 g fat, 2 mg cholesterol, 3 g fiber, 79 mg sodium, 221 mg calcium

Chocolate Egg Cream*

Try this delicious old-fashioned treat when you want something sweet and fizzy.

1 tablespoon chocolate syrup
6 ounces 1% milk
6 ounces seltzer

In a tall glass, stir together the chocolate syrup, milk, and seltzer.

Serves 1

Per serving: 125 calories, 2 g fat, 8 mg cholesterol, 0 mg fiber, 159 mg sodium, 159 mg calcium

Island Shake

In this recipe, mangoes and bananas combine to create a rich, creamy texture.

1 can (8 ounces) juice-packed pineapple chunks
1 cup sliced or chopped peeled fresh or prepared mango
1 ripe banana, sliced
1 cup fat-free vanilla frozen yogurt
Crushed or cracked ice

In a blender, combine the pineapple (with juice), mango, and banana. Process until smooth. Add the frozen yogurt. Blend well.

With the blender running, gradually drop in enough ice to bring the level up to 4 cups. Blend until the ice is pureed.

Serves 4

Per serving: 142 calories, 0.3 g fat, 0 mg cholesterol, 2.1 g fiber, 37 mg sodium, 62 mg calcium

Note: Look for jars of prepared mango slices in the refrigerated section of the produce department or bags of chopped mango in the freezer section.

Peach Smoothie*

Peaches and cinnamon lend a touch of sweetness to this satisfying smoothie.

*1 large ripe peach, peeled and sliced; 1 cup diced peach
   canned in juice; or 1 cup frozen peach slices*
1 tablespoon sugar
1 cup fat-free vanilla ice cream
1/2 cup orange juice
Pinch of ground cinnamon

In a blender, combine the peach and sugar. Add the ice cream, orange juice, and cinnamon. Blend until smooth.
Serves 2
Per serving: 236 calories, 0 g fat, 5 mg cholesterol, 2 g fiber, 81 mg sodium, 109 mg calcium

Cantaloupe Cooler

This just might be the perfect drink for a summer brunch.

2 cups cantaloupe cubes
1 ripe banana, sliced
1/2 cup fat-free vanilla yogurt
1/2 cup orange juice
4 ice cubes, cracked

Combine the cantaloupe, banana, yogurt, orange juice, and ice cubes in a blender. Process until smooth. Pour into tall glasses.
Serves 3
Per serving: 121 calories, 0.6 g fat, 1 mg cholesterol, 1.8 g fiber, 34 mg sodium, 85 mg calcium

Chocolate Malted*

Who can resist this classic soda-fountain favorite?

1 1/2 cups fat-free chocolate ice cream
1/2 cup fat-free milk
4 1/2 tablespoons chocolate malted milk powder

In a blender, combine the ice cream, milk, and malted milk powder. Blend until smooth.
Serves 2
Per serving: 340 calories, 3 g fat, 5 mg cholesterol, 2 g fiber, 234 mg sodium, 443 mg calcium
Note: Look for chocolate malted milk powder in the coffee aisle of your supermarket.

Icy Mango Shiver*
Whip up this creamy tropical concoction in minutes using prepared mango slices.

$\frac{1}{2}$ cup sliced or chopped peeled fresh or prepared mango
1 tablespoon sugar
$\frac{3}{4}$ cup fat-free vanilla yogurt
$\frac{1}{2}$ cup crushed ice

Place the mango, sugar, yogurt, and ice in a blender and whirl until smooth. Serve immediately.
Serves 2
Per serving: 150 calories, 0 g fat, 0 mg cholesterol, 1 g fiber, 52 mg sodium, 155 mg calcium
Note: Look for jars of prepared mango slices in the refrigerated section of the produce department or bags of chopped mango in the freezer section.

Dreamy Orange Cream*
Frozen yogurt makes this frosty drink extra-easy.

3 cups orange juice
2 cups fat-free vanilla frozen yogurt
2 tablespoons all-fruit orange marmalade
6 ice cubes, cracked
Mint leaves

In a blender, combine the orange juice, frozen yogurt, marmalade, and ice cubes. Process until smooth. Pour into tall glasses. Garnish with the mint.
Serves 4

Per serving: 205 calories, 0.4 g fat, 0 mg cholesterol, 1.5 g fiber, 72 mg sodium, 120 mg calcium

Kiwi Cooler*

Somehow "delicious" doesn't seem to do this drink justice. It's super-easy, too!

2 kiwifruit, peeled and sliced
4 cups fat-free vanilla frozen yogurt

In a food processor or blender, combine the kiwifruit and frozen yogurt. Process until smooth. Serve in tall glasses.

Serves 4

Per serving: 214 calories, 0.5 g fat, 3 mg cholesterol, 0.7 g fiber, 131 mg sodium, 210 mg calcium

CHAPTER FOURTEEN

Almost Everyone Can Scream for Ice Cream

Maybe you think the Ice Cream Diet isn't for you because you have diabetes and you can't eat sugar. Or you have lactose intolerance and you can't digest milk properly. Or you are allergic to milk, or at least suspect you are.

Well, I've got wonderful news for you. According to experts in the medical specialties that deal with these conditions, just about anyone can eat ice cream! The key is to understand your particular condition, so you're prepared to make any necessary adjustments in the Ice Cream Diet. Then you can throw away your worries!

So allow me to give you the scoop on a trio of health problems that at first blush might seem incompatible with the Ice Cream Diet. I'll show you what you can do to enjoy the requisite serving of ice cream (or another frozen treat) every day. By the time I'm done, I suspect you'll be poised with your spoon!

IF YOU HAVE A MILK ALLERGY . . .

If personal perceptions are any indication, milk allergies are rampant in this country. An estimated 30 percent of the U.S. population believes they are allergic to milk. "But contrary to popular belief, most adults do not have milk allergies," notes Anne Muñoz-Furlong, founder and president of The Food Allergy and Anaphylaxis Network in Fairfax, Virginia. In fact, only about 2 percent of those who suspect they have milk allergies actually do.

How do you know if you're one of the few who truly need to keep milk off the menu? First, be aware that milk allergy—an immune reaction to the protein in dairy products, including ice cream—is much more common in children than in adults. What's more, about 85 percent of children grow out of this allergy by about age 3.

And once you're an adult, milk allergy seldom appears out of the blue, unlike the more common food allergies to shellfish and peanuts. In other words, if you haven't had a milk allergy since you were a kid, you're unlikely to develop one as an adult.

In a true milk allergy, the symptoms usually occur within minutes of eating a dairy product. Most common is some form of skin rash; you may develop hives, red blotches, and itching anywhere on your body. A skin reaction might be accompanied by digestive symptoms, such as cramps, vomiting, and diarrhea. Respiratory problems—including difficulty breathing and swelling of the throat, tongue, and lips—have been reported, too.

Such symptoms are nothing to toy with. "Sometimes when they're left untreated, they trigger a more serious reaction that can be life threatening," Muñoz-Furlong notes. So if you suspect you have a true milk allergy, see a physician who is a board-certified allergist specializing in food-related reactions.

Those who have true milk allergies cannot eat ice cream or other foods made from milk or milk components, including casein and whey protein. But even if you are one of the few who must steer clear of ice cream, you can still slim down on the Ice Cream Diet! In "Fabulous Fakes" at right, you'll read about some amazing nondairy frozen desserts that can be substituted for ice cream safely and deliciously.

You will need to make sure you're getting enough calcium from nondairy sources. Look for fortified orange juice

FABULOUS FAKES

Can't eat ice cream that comes from a cow? Or just don't want to? Don't despair. Supermarkets and health-food stores have never been so flush with nondairy frozen desserts as they are today.

Most of these products are marketed for the lactose intolerant, says Cynthia Sass, R.D., a registered dietitian in Tampa, Florida, and a spokeswoman for the American Dietetic Association. They're sold under brand names like Tofutti, Soy Delicious, Better Than Ice Cream, and DariFree*ze. "The products are comparable to ice cream," Sass says. And most are dairy-free. Many are made from soy, while others are based on rice, oats, and even potato.

Read labels for calorie content; to qualify for the Ice Cream Diet, a nondairy frozen dessert should supply no more than 125 calories per serving. Check labels for calcium too, Sass advises. Some products—especially those made from soy—are calcium fortified. Others may not meet the calcium guidelines for the Ice Cream Diet. Ideally, they should offer about 100 milligrams, or 10 percent of the Daily Value, per 1/2-cup serving.

Some studies have suggested that you absorb less calcium from soy products than from dairy. "The bottom line is, we don't absorb a whole lot of calcium at any one time, no matter where it comes from—food or supplement," Sass says. Spread your calcium throughout the day, she advises, and you'll benefit most.

Another tip for finding dairy-free frozen desserts? Choose kosher products, suggests Daryl Altman, M.D., an allergist, immunologist, and researcher in Baldwin, New York. They shouldn't contain even a hint of dairy. To be sure, look for the word "pareve" on the label.

In nonkosher foods, check ingredient lists for the words "casein" and "whey protein." These milk compounds turn up in many foods you may not think of as dairy products. "You must be a good label reader," Dr. Altman says.

and tomato juice, fortified cereals, and fortified soy milks. A calcium supplement might help, too.

To learn more about milk allergy, visit www.food allergy.org, the official Web site of the Food Allergy and Anaphylaxis Network. Or call the organization's toll-free number: (800) 929–4040.

IF YOU CAN'T DIGEST MILK . . .

According to Muñoz-Furlong, many people confuse milk allergy with milk intolerance. In fact, the two conditions are very different.

While milk allergy is relatively rare, milk intolerance is considered quite common. Also known as lactose intolerance, this condition affects up to 75 percent of people worldwide. Those of dark-skinned ethnicities seem especially vulnerable, while those of Scandinavian or more northern ancestry are seldom affected.

While milk intolerance is bothersome, it isn't life threatening. And it shouldn't prevent you from enjoying ice cream!

If you have milk intolerance, you lack the digestive enzyme *lactase*, which breaks down a special type of sugar found in milk called *lactose*. When we are born, virtually all of us have the ability to digest lactose. After all, mother's milk is the first food infants eat, so they must have plenty of lactase to thrive. But as we get older, the lactase in the intestine decreases to a greater or lesser degree. The more it decreases, the more trouble you'll have.

Symptoms of lactose intolerance can emerge within a half-hour to 2 hours of eating dairy products, including ice cream, says Leslie Bonci, R.D., director of sports nutrition at the University of Pittsburgh Medical Center. The undigested milk sugar travels to the large intestine, where it ferments. Unlike milk allergy, lactose intolerance causes *only* gastrointestinal distress, including gas, bloating, diarrhea, and stomach upset. It doesn't trigger rashes or breathing problems.

What's surprising is, most people with lactose intolerance experience almost no noticeable symptoms at all, save for some mild gas that is imperceptible to others. Says Bonci: "What people sometimes think is lactose intolerance actually is lactose maldigestion, a milder version of the condition."

In fact, even those whose symptoms are more pronounced likely won't suffer any consequences from eating a serving of ice cream a day (1 cup for women, 1½ cups for men). That's provided the ice cream doesn't follow a dairy-rich meal, such as lasagna or macaroni and cheese.

Research has shown that consuming up to 12 grams of lactose per serving—probably more than you'd get from your daily ice cream treat—produces virtually no symptoms of lactose intolerance, says Michael Levitt, M.D., associate chief of staff at the University of Minnesota School of Medicine Veterans Affairs Medical Center and a specialist in the condition. In one small study involving 21 African-American girls between ages 11 and 15, symptoms were "negligible" even after 3 weeks on a high-dairy diet.

If eating even ½ cup of ice cream triggers your gastrointestinal symptoms, Bonci suggests trying 2 tablespoons and gradually working your way up to 8—the equivalent of ½ cup. Then keep going until you're able to eat your full serving of ice cream every day. "Most people (with lactose intolerance) can learn to tolerate dairy foods," Bonci says.

Another option is to try supplemental lactase enzymes. They're available over the counter as chewable tablets. Start taking them according to the label directions, Bonci says, and increase the dosage as necessary. The tablets are perfectly safe. Just be sure to take them 20 to 30 minutes *before* you eat your ice cream. "After is too late," Bonci cautions.

If your symptoms persist, see your doctor. Researchers report that what some patients describe as lactose intolerance actually is irritable bowel syndrome, Dr. Levitt says.

WHAT ABOUT THE "OTHER" MILK ALLERGY?

Despite the fact that few people are actually allergic to milk, thousands seem convinced they are—and scores of books blame milk for a host of ailments. One of the most common complaints? That milk and other dairy products cause the respiratory passages to produce mucus that leads to a stuffy nose and coughing. Other complaints cite dairy as a factor in everything from headache to back pain to fatigue.

Experts like Daryl Altman, M.D., an allergist and immunologist in Baldwin, New York, say double-blind, placebo-controlled studies—considered the gold standard in scientific research—just don't support these charges against milk. Nevertheless, Dr. Altman's own studies have identified milk as one of the two foods that people, especially women, most commonly perceive as triggering adverse reactions. (The other is chocolate!) What's going on here?

In general, Dr. Altman says, most people lack understanding of food allergies. "Because we eat anywhere from three to six times per day, any event in our lives will be close to some meal," she explains. "So it's very easy to assume that, say, your headache is caused by something you ate an hour ago."

"People tend to describe any symptom related to a food as an allergy," Dr. Altman adds. "A person who experiences diarrhea from food poisoning may never eat that particular food again, assuming it's an 'allergy.' Or if a person eats a spicy meal close to bedtime and wakes up with heartburn, again, it must be 'allergy.'"

Even skin rashes are routinely attributed to milk allergy, almost as a knee-jerk reaction, Dr. Altman observes. In fact, a rash can be a symptom of a host of ailments, including viral infection, heat rash, anxiety, lupus, lymphoma, and hepatitis.

Part of the reason milk has been blamed for respiratory symptoms like coughing may be that some adults experience the texture of milk as somewhat slimy, Muñoz-Furlong says. The same could be true for ice cream: People might be mistaking the slimy sensation for mucus, she speculates.

Then, too, milk is so prominent in the American diet that it's easily singled out as a problem food. People know that babies can be allergic to cow's milk, Dr. Altman says. So they assume that adults can be allergic, too. "And they believe that they can diagnose milk allergy on their own," Dr. Altman adds. "So that's what they do: They self-diagnose."

Still, if you're absolutely convinced that milk is behind a particular symptom or ailment that you've been experiencing, try eliminating dairy products from your diet for a week or two. If your symptoms disappear while you're dairy-free, then start thinking about how you can get enough calcium from fortified foods like orange juice and soy milk. And see

---

BEATING "BRAIN FREEZE"

If you eat ice cream quickly or gulp a cold drink, you might experience a sudden rush of pain to your forehead and temples. Known as a cold stimulus headache, the pain peaks within 25 to 60 seconds and may last for as long as 5 minutes.

Not many people get this sort of headache, says Seymour Diamond, M.D., director of the Diamond Headache Clinic in Chicago and executive chairman of the National Headache Foundation. In fact, estimates are that only about one-third of us do.

These people have sensitive nerves in the palate and the pharynx, Dr. Diamond explains. When stimulated, these nerves send pain signals to the brain.

More than 90 percent of people who get migraines report that they also experience ice cream headache. While an ice cream headache could trigger a migraine, it usually will not, Dr. Diamond says. Similarly, if you get migraines, you may never experience ice cream headache at all.

You might be able to beat what professional ice cream taster John Harrison of Edy's Grand Ice Cream in Oakland, California, calls brain freeze by letting your ice cream temper for several minutes before digging in. Most important, says Dr. Diamond: "Don't gulp your ice cream." (Well, we can try!)

"Fabulous Fakes" on page 175 for nondairy frozen desserts that fit within the framework of the Ice Cream Diet.

IF YOU HAVE DIABETES . . .

Not all that long ago, people who had diabetes were routinely told they could not eat sugar. And ice cream, which is sweetened with sugar, was one of many foods considered

---

THE MILK CONTROVERSY

Who says men and milk don't mix?

The animal-rights group PETA (People for the Ethical Treatment of Animals), for one. Perhaps you've seen some of their scary ads saying that milk causes prostate cancer. The group bases its warnings on a 2001 study at Harvard University and Brigham and Women's Hospital in Boston linking calcium to prostate cancer.

But before any guy gives up calcium, he'd best take a closer look at the study's findings. For 11 years, researchers followed 20,855 men, 1,012 of whom developed prostate cancer. According to Peter Holt, M.D., a cancer specialist at St. Luke's–Roosevelt Hospital in New York City, the only suggestion of a relationship between calcium and prostate cancer was among about 16 subjects whose calcium intakes exceeded 2,500 milligrams a day. (That's extremely high—far more than a guy would get from the Ice Cream Diet.) The small number of subjects in that highest-calcium group makes drawing accurate conclusions difficult.

What's more, Dr. Holt says, "the men who were getting a more normal amount of calcium, about 1,000 milligrams, saw no negative effect. And they were the largest group in the study."

While the Harvard researchers suggest that more research is needed to establish a link between calcium and cancer, they note that men need calcium to help prevent any thinning of their bones as they age. Guys still should aim for their suggested calcium intake of 1,000 to 1,500 milligrams a day.

off-limits, says Anne Daly, R.D., president of health care and education for the American Diabetes Association, based in Alexandria, Virginia.

Today, the rule book is not so rigid. If you have diabetes, you *can* eat sugar. And you can follow the Ice Cream Diet!

"For some time, the American Diabetes Association has advised that sugar can be part of a healthy diet," Daly says. In fact, today we know that inside your body, the carbohydrate in sugar has the same effect on blood sugar levels as the carbohydrate in starches such as bread and potatoes.

"If you have diabetes, you need to monitor your total intake of carbohydrates, one of which is sugar," Daly explains. "We set carbohydrate targets. If you eat ice cream, for example, you need to be sure it fits within your carbohydrate count for the day. That's very individual, and it's very important for fine-tuning blood sugar control."

A registered dietitian can play a pivotal role in teaching you how to incorporate foods with sugar into a healthy diet. I suggest that if you have diabetes and would like to try the Ice Cream Diet, you work with your dietitian to make sure she knows about the eating plan you intend to follow. Above all, please don't simply add a bowl of ice cream to the eating plan you're already on.

One aspect of the Ice Cream Diet that makes it ideal for people with diabetes is its emphasis on healthy, balanced meals and snacks featuring a bounty of fruits and vegetables—at least eight servings a day! "Fruits and vegetables are especially important for people with diabetes, and that's the area where most Americans have some work to do," Daly notes.

What else makes the Ice Cream Diet especially good for people with diabetes? Its controlled calories help melt away excess pounds. That's important because some 80 percent of people with type 2 diabetes are overweight, and the number is climbing, Daly says. If you have diabetes, losing even 5 to 7 percent of your current body weight can reduce your risks of complications from the disease.

Ironically, among the foods that people with diabetes can

be lulled into overeating are the so-called no-sugar-added treats. These products, which sometimes are labeled "sugar-free," get their sweetness not from sugar but from lower-calorie substitutes like maltitol, a sugar alcohol. "The problem is that many diabetics assume 'no sugar added' or 'sugar-free' means zero calories," Daly says. "And that's definitely not always true."

Many calories in these products, including no-sugar-added ice cream, can come from fat as well as from some of the lower-calorie sweeteners and bulking agents that replace sugar. In fact, some sugar-free versions of treats like ice cream or cookies have as many or nearly as many calories as products sweetened with sugar! But unless you look carefully for the calories on the label, you could be deceived into eating way too much.

People with diabetes *can* work some sugar into a balanced, calorie-controlled diet, Daly says. In fact, having that sugar, in sensible amounts, may be to your advantage when you're following a healthy eating plan like the Ice Cream Diet.

"Food needs to be enjoyed," Daly explains. "If having some sugar adds pleasure and satisfaction to your meals, you're more likely to stick with the healthy diet that's so important if you have diabetes."

So eat your ice cream in moderation—and enjoy!

PART V

Exercise Your Right to Slim Down

CHAPTER FIFTEEN

Every Reason to Shape Up

It's deceptively simple. To lose weight, you can either eat fewer calories than your body needs or burn off calories with exercise. The easiest and most effective way to lose weight is to combine the two methods. Here's why. To lose a pound of fat, you need to eliminate 3,500 calories. Cutting that many from your diet, however, even spread out over a week, can be really tough. Food just tastes too good. Similarly, burning all those calories with exercise alone is a tall order. Since walking a mile burns about 80 calories, you'd have to trek for 44 miles to lose a pound!

So losing weight is easier if you combine calorie cutting *and* exercise. To lose about a pound a week, you need a 500-calorie deficit each day. You can achieve that by cutting calories (on the Ice Cream Diet, you'll be eating 300 to 500 fewer calories a day than you normally would) and by exercising (a 2-mile walk burns about 150 calories).

If images of fanatical aerobics instructors or muscle-bound weight lifters pop into your mind when you think of exercise, relax. It's a common misconception that exercise only works if it hurts. For example, almost half of the visitors to *Prevention*'s Web site imagine exercise as longer, tougher, or more frequent than it needs to be.

The truth is, you *can* lose fat without breaking a sweat. By accumulating each day 30 minutes of activities such as cleaning your home and walking to the video store instead of driving, you can yield the same results as taking aerobics classes 3 days a week. Even squeezing in 10 minutes of walking several times throughout your day adds up to pounds off.

YOUR BASIC EXERCISE PRESCRIPTION

When you're just starting out, *Prevention* recommends that you aim for 30 minutes of aerobic exercise, 3 to 5 days a week, and 20 minutes of strength training, 2 to 3 days a week. Pretty soon, however, for weight loss (and to maintain your weight once you reach your goal), you need to bump that moderate aerobic activity up to 45 to 60 minutes at least five times a week. The recommendation for strength training becomes 20 to 30 minutes, 2 to 3 days a week.

Experts caution beginner exercisers against jumping into vigorous exercise programs. If you're just starting out, beginning with a demanding running program isn't practical, safe, or likely sustainable. Instead, moderate intensity and duration work best. Simply do whatever gets you moving regularly.

EXCUSE-PROOF YOUR WORKOUT

So, what *does* get you moving regularly? Or, more important, what keeps you from moving regularly? Here's how to combat your strongest exercise excuses.

"I don't think I can exercise." Take a dose of positive thinking. Self-perception has a strong influence on physical performance, experts say. To get yourself going, surround yourself with positive people, and do things that make you feel confident.

"I don't have time to exercise." Look at your life and evaluate what's important to you. People just as busy as you are find time to exercise. When you make exercise a priority, you make time for it.

"I feel out of place when I exercise." Join a class designed for a wide range of exercisers. It will be a more com-

fortable and fun environment. To locate a class, check your local YM/YWCA, churches, colleges, and gyms.

"I don't like how I look." Go shopping! You can look and feel great if you choose the right clothes. Women, for example, can purchase stylish, supportive active wear in sizes 14 and up from Junonia. Call (800) 586–6642 or visit www.junonia.com for a free catalog.

"I get bored exercising." It's easy to get into an exercise rut and walk around the same blocks, day after day after day. The two chapters that follow offer dozens of different, fun exercises to try. Plus, keep in mind that there are two main types of exercise: aerobic exercise (movement that gets your heart pumping and burns fat, such as walking and cycling) and strength training or weight-bearing exercise (movement that builds shapely muscles and revs your metabolism to burn more calories, such as weight lifting and calisthenics). The best exercise program includes both aerobic conditioning and strength training, providing instant variety. You'll learn more about aerobic exercise in chapter 16 and strength training in chapter 17.

"I'm not motivated to exercise." For many people, the promise of weight loss is reason enough to get moving. Other people, however, need several incentives. If you still lack motivation even after imagining your slim and toned body, read on to learn about the many healthy benefits of exercise.

EXERCISE MAKES *EVERYTHING* BETTER

Regular exercise has dozens of benefits—for both your body and your mind. Take a look at just a few of them.

- Migraine prevention. Any form of aerobic exercise may help prevent the crushing pain of migraines. Exercise stimulates the body to release endorphins, brain chemicals that improve mood. Exercise also helps to relieve stress, one of the known headache triggers.
- Heart protection. Like all muscles, your heart becomes stronger and more efficient with exercise. Activity actually protects against heart attacks.

BURN OFF A SPLURGE? YOU BE THE JUDGE

On the Ice Cream Diet, you can indulge in a nice-size dish of ice cream every day and still lose weight. That's the beauty of this plan. But what if you order one of those go-for-broke sundaes, the kind you hope no one notices the waiter is delivering to *your* table? Do you secretly promise that you'll wipe out all those extra calories with exercise?

Okay, let's do some math and see how realistic that is. The point, here, is not that you can *never* splurge. But splurging often and thinking you'll exercise those calories away? Not a chance. As an example, let's take that foot-high, chocolate-dripping, whipped-cream-topped Reese's Peanut Butter Cup sundae with 930 calories. Here's how many minutes the average 150-pound woman would have to exercise to burn off this splurge.

EXERCISE	CALORIES BURNED PER MINUTE	NUMBER OF MINUTES TO BURN OFF A SUNDAE
Aerobics	7.4	126
Backpacking	7.9	118
Bicycling	9.1	102
Calisthenics	9.1	102
Cleaning	3.4	274
Dancing	5.1	182
Gardening	4.5	207
Ice-skating	7.9	118
Jogging	7.9	118
Jumping rope	9.1	102
Snowshoeing	9.1	102
Swimming	7.9	118
Tai chi	4.5	207
Tennis	7.9	118
Walking	4.4	211
Yoga	2.8	332

• Cholesterol reduction. Exercise helps your cholesterol in two ways. First, it raises HDL, the good cholesterol. Second, it reduces LDL cholesterol, the bad kind that forms artery-clogging plaque and contributes to high blood pressure, heart attacks, and strokes.

• Diabetes prevention. Exercise can prevent diabetes or help control it if you already have it. Working out enables muscles to take up blood sugar and use it as energy, helping keep blood sugar and insulin levels on an even keel.

• Stronger bones. Strength training helps maintain or even increase bone density. Lifetime walkers are less likely to develop osteoporosis.

• Colon cancer prevention. Exercise speeds the movement of digested food through the colon, denying potential carcinogens the opportunity to affect the colon lining.

• Boosted immunity. Exercise offers powerful protection against colds and flu. One study found that those who exercised for just 20 minutes a day were significantly less likely to call in sick from work than nonexercisers.

• Breast cancer protection. By reducing body fat, exercise reduces the production of estrogen, which promotes some kinds of breast cancer.

• Pain relief. Exercise is nature's aspirin. In one study, a 25-minute spin on a stationary bike significantly reduced the level of back pain felt by eight people. And, the relief lasted for up to ½ hour after they stopped pedaling.

• Mood improvement. Exercise rids the body of stress hormones, brightening mood and relieving feelings of depression and anxiety. Most people feel a sense of calm and well-being after a workout. Think of a runner's high, for example.

• Less stress. Any exercise can reduce stress. It helps relieve muscle tension and sends oxygenated blood to the brain and other vital organs.

• Better self-esteem. In one study, researchers found that regular light to moderate activity improves self-esteem. Even stretching and toning helped. They found a signifi-

TALK WITH YOUR DOCTOR

If you have a chronic condition or are clinically obese (defined as exceeding a healthy weight by 30 percent or more), check with your doctor before beginning any exercise program.

When you get the go-ahead, here are some tips for exercising if you have one of the following health conditions.

HIGH BLOOD PRESSURE OR OTHER HEART CONDITIONS

Regular exercise is beneficial for people with heart conditions. Studies show that regular exercise lowers blood pressure by an average of 10 points. Plus, exercise helps weight loss, which also lowers blood pressure.

To work out safely with high blood pressure, exercise moderately, lift carefully (using a moderate, not heavy, weight), stand up slowly after stretching or exercising on the floor, and work out daily. The best exercises for people with high blood pressure are walking and weight lifting.

If you are taking blood pressure medicine that controls your heart rate, do not overexert when exercising. With some medicines, your pulse will not increase, but your blood pressure will rise. Don't hold your breath when exercising. This can put a strain on your heart.

OSTEOPOROSIS AND LOW BONE DENSITY

Regular exercise lowers the risk of osteoporosis by strengthening bones. It is especially helpful in strengthening the bones of the hip area. To work out safely with osteoporosis, first get a bone-density test and find out from your doctor which activities may be risky for you. When exercising, you may need more rest while strength training. Take a 1- to 2-minute break between exercises and allow 2 days of rest between strength-training workouts. Avoid exercises that require you to bend your back forward. It's safe to bend forward from the hips if you keep your back straight. Skip sports that are high impact or involve risk of falling. If your coordination is poor, use treadmills only if they have sturdy handrails.

The best exercises for people with osteoporosis are walking and gardening. Jumping jacks, tennis, swing dance, and step aerobics are great, too, because they're higher impact and strengthen bones. Tai chi and strength training are also good because strong muscles and good balance prevent falls. To order the exercise video "Be BoneWise Exercise," which was designed for women with osteoporosis, visit the National Osteoporosis Foundation Web site at www.nof.org.

CANCER

Regular exercise is linked with lower cancer risk. Plus, exercise helps with weight loss. Experts say that maintaining a healthy weight is key to cancer prevention.

If you have been diagnosed with cancer, talk with your doctor for information specific to your condition.

In general, though, while doctors used to advise people with cancer to rest, now they recommend exercise. In some studies, people with cancer who did moderate exercise reported decreased nausea, decreased fatigue, increased physical tolerance for activity, and increased quality of life. Aerobic exercise that increases the heart rate increased red blood cell production and improved the functioning of the heart, lungs, and circulation.

If you have cancer, don't exercise if your blood counts are low or if you're at risk for infection, anemia, or bleeding. Also, don't exercise if the level of minerals in your blood, such as sodium and potassium, are not normal. Avoid uneven surfaces or excessive weight-bearing exercises, which could result in a fall and injury.

Don't exercise if you have unrelieved pain, nausea or vomiting, or any other symptom that causes you concern.

cant decrease in self-esteem when people stopped exercising.

• Wintertime blues reduction. Many people experience some degree of seasonal affective disorder or wintertime depression. Exercise is a natural antidepressant. But just like antidepressants, it needs to be taken daily.

• Energy production. It seems counterintuitive, but expending energy through exercise actually *increases* energy. For one reason, the fitter you are, the less energy it takes you to do everyday tasks. Plus even activities like walking from the car into the grocery store offer immediate energy boosts by pumping oxygenated blood through your body.

• Better sleep. Studies show that fit people sleep better, fall asleep quicker, wake up less often, and experience more deep sleep.

• Quicker reaction time. Stereotypes suggest that the older we get, the slower we move. Research shows that you can actually prevent the decline of reaction time and stay sharp through exercise.

• A career boost. No kidding. In one study, researchers discovered that people who exercised were rated as harder workers and more attractive, healthy, and in control than nonexercisers or people whose exercise habits were unknown.

• More money! Exercise can even boost your financial fitness by lowering medical bills. When researchers reviewed the medical costs of active people and compared them with those of inactive people, they found that overall adults who exercised saved $330 a year in medical expenses such as doctor visits, hospitalization, and medication.

• A longer life. Not only does exercise add life to your years, it adds years to your life. Researchers who assessed the muscle strength of more than 8,000 people for 20 years found that those who could do the most curl-ups were more likely to be alive at the study's end than those who did the least. Another study found that exercising vigorously three times a week can add 2.1 years to your life span!

Now get moving!

CHAPTER SIXTEEN

Walk, Run, or Bike to Your Ice Cream Cone

Here's a great way to motivate yourself to get moving. Think of exercise as currency. Extra exercise buys you extra food. If, for example, you walk ½ hour at a moderate pace to and from the ice cream shop, you'll have burned off the 250 calories in your cup of reduced-calorie ice cream!

Activities like walking, running, or biking are known as aerobic, or cardio, exercise. This type of exercise conditions your heart and lungs, helps lower cholesterol and control blood pressure, fights diabetes, and improves your endurance. As mentioned in chapter 15, *Prevention* recommends that you aim for 45 to 60 minutes of moderate aerobic activity at least five times a week in order to lose weight and—*most important*—to keep off the weight once you've lost it.

If you're a fitness newbie, here's a fabulous aerobic workout to get you moving safely. It lets you work up gradually to your 45-minute daily minimum. This super-easy fitness-walking plan provides maximum benefits without injury, alternating moderate walking and brisk walking. Do at least 5 minutes of easy walking before you start and a few minutes of stretching to warm up and cool down. At the end of your walk, you should feel mildly tired, not exhausted. Under normal circumstances, take 2 days off during each

The Beginner's *Prevention* Aerobic Workout

	DAY 1 TEMPO	DAY 2 BUMP IT UP	DAY 3 LONG	DAY 4 TEMPO	DAY 5 1-MINUTE COUNT
WEEK 1	15 minutes	20 minutes	30 minutes	15 minutes	20 minutes
WEEK 2	20 minutes	25 minutes	30 minutes	20 minutes	25 minutes
WEEK 3	15 minutes	25 minutes	30 minutes	15 minutes	25 minutes
WEEK 4	20 minutes	25 minutes	35 minutes	20 minutes	25 minutes

Key

Tempo/Long: Walk at a moderate pace that's brisk enough to get your heart pumping but that won't leave you out of breath.

Bump It Up: Walk for 5 minutes at a moderate pace, then speed up for 1 minute. Repeat for the total time.

1-Minute Count: Walk for 5 minutes at a moderate pace, then count the number of steps you take for 1 minute. Repeat for the total time. The satisfaction here is, as you get faster, the number of steps will increase.

week. But if you need to, skip a day or scale back on the number of minutes.

Once you've mastered the 4-week start-up program, it's important to bump up the duration of your walks to 45 to 60 minutes, 5 or more days a week. Or add other aerobic activities so that you reach that very important 45- to 60-minute daily total.

AEROBIC TIPS

One reason this fitness-walking workout is so effective is that it uses interval training. Performing tougher bouts of exercise followed by easier ones may burn fat faster than working out at a steady pace. This type of "rest and go" training helps beat boredom and fatigue, too.

In one study, one group of exercisers worked out 5 days a week at a steady rate for up to 45 minutes. Another group exercised for the same amount of time, but they varied their

Exercise—Beyond Walking

ACTIVITY	CALORIES BURNED*	BIGGEST BENEFIT	FUN FACTOR
Agility training with your dog	204	Builds strong legs and improves cardio fitness.	Training with your dog is both invigorating and relaxing.
Bicycling	238	Tones butt and leg muscles.	Flying down hills is still fun.
Bowling	102	Burn about three times as many calories as watching TV.	It's a great activity for the entire family.
Canoeing	335	Strengthens shoulders, arms, back, and abdominals.	Discover interesting wildlife and beautiful scenery.
Gardening	136	Second only to lifting weights as the top bone preserver.	Get a workout *and* a beautiful yard.
Golf	153	Decreases abdominal fat and increases endurance.	It's a fun excuse to hang out with friends.
Jazz dancing	163	This high-impact exercise is good for your bones and improves posture.	Makes you feel sexy.

Exercise—Beyond Walking (cont.)

ACTIVITY	CALORIES BURNED*	BIGGEST BENEFIT	FUN FACTOR
Jumping Rope	272	Tones your hips, thighs, and butt. Great bone builder, too.	Requires total concentra- tion—block out all your worries.
Mall walking	130	A great way to strengthen yourheart and increase lung power.	It's the perfect excuse to window-shop.
Playground fun	150	Strengthens legs,arms, and butt.	Your kids will delight in swinging, seesawing, and sliding with you.
Rebounding	150	Increases circulation, and coordination.	Encourages you to jump around like a maniac.
Skipping	170	Works your legs and provides a good cardio workout. Builds bone, too.	It's like being a kid again.
Softball	170	Speeds reaction time and sharpens hand/eye coordination.	Savor the sound when bat and ball connect— whack!

Exercise—Beyond Walking (cont.)

ACTIVITY	CALORIES BURNED*	BIGGEST BENEFIT	FUN FACTOR
Speed skating	306	Tones your butt, thighs, legs, and abs.	Feed your need for speed!
Speed walking (5 mph or faster, 12-minute mile)	272	Burns more calories and boosts fitness faster than jogging at the same speed.	It's a thrill to walk "in the fast lane."
Stairclimbing	204	Great for toning muscle and building bone.	Picture yourself in Philadelphia and hum the theme to *Rocky*.
Swimming	272	Easy on the joints and works practically every muscle in your body.	You don't sweat in the water!
Tennis	238	Improves arm, shoulder, and leg strength and flattens your belly.	Helps you understand the U.S. Open—and John McEnroe.

Exercise—Beyond Walking (cont.)

ACTIVITY	CALORIES BURNED*	BIGGEST BENEFIT	FUN FACTOR
Trail walking	129	Builds bones and improves lower body strength.	Bring along binoculars for bird-watching to take you to a new world of adventure.
Walking in water	170	Improves lower body strength (think prettier legs!).	The weightless feeling makes you feel as though you're in outer space.
Yoga	85	Keeps muscles and joints strong and flexible.	Brings you peace and quiet!

*Calories burned are for the average 150-pound woman, exercising for 30 minutes.

intensity. After 10 weeks, the "rest and go" group lost more than three times the weight of the continuous exercisers.

To keep yourself motivated and make exercise more fun, it helps to have lots of exercises from which to choose. Think of it as your fitness smorgasbord. Trying new exercises helps you get fit faster, beat boredom, and avoid injury. Fun activities don't feel like exercise, but they do burn calories.

CHAPTER SEVENTEEN

Lift More Than Your Spoon

An exercise program with just aerobic exercise and no strength training is like a peanut butter sandwich with no jelly. It's good, but not as great as it could be.

The best exercise programs combine aerobic conditioning *and* strength training. Both types of exercise are important for different reasons. Aerobic exercise conditions your heart and lungs, helps lower cholesterol and blood pressure levels, and improves your endurance. But strength training—which is also called weight training, resistance training, or weight lifting—helps prevent the loss of muscle that usually occurs as you age. Examples of strength training are lifting free weights like dumbbells, working out on gym weight machines, and even calisthenics like pushups and situps.

Strength training is important because as you age, unless you use your muscles, you automatically lose them—more and more every year. The great news is, if you work your major muscle groups twice a week, you can expect to replace 5 to 10 years' worth of muscle loss in just a few months! It's like turning back the hands of time, or rolling back the odometer in your body's motor. Lifting weights can literally reverse the aging process, so you look and feel years, maybe even decades, younger.

If you're a woman who's worried about looking like Mr. Universe, delete that worry from your list. Unless you're lifting major weights for hours a day, all you'll get are sleek, taut muscles that only make you look sexy and trim. There's a *reason* that so many models and actresses have started lifting weights!

Lifting weights even helps you fight the battle of the bulge *while you sleep*! That is not a fairy tale but basic science: Resistance training builds muscle, and muscles burn considerably more calories per hour than fat. Here's the simple math. To sustain a pound of fat for a day, your body spends a measly 2 calories. By contrast, sustaining a pound of muscle for a day requires 30 calories. Let's say that you exercise faithfully and replace 2 pounds of fat with 2 pounds of muscle. That means every day, even while you watch *Friends* or *Law & Order*, surf the Internet, and sleep, your body burns as many as 60 extra calories just to keep you alive. Within a year, you'd lose more than 6 pounds.

In addition to preserving—and increasing—your muscles, strength training also preserves—and builds—your bones. This is critical for people trying to lose weight. An insidious side effect of dieting is that when you cut calories too drastically, in addition to losing body fat, you also lose muscle and bone. In one study, women who lost an average of 7 pounds also lost significant bone-mineral density in the process. Strength training combats this loss.

And yet there's more. Another benefit to adding strength training to aerobic exercise is that the combination boosts mood even more than aerobics alone. Experts suspect that strength training makes people feel strong and independent. Aerobic activity boosts feel-good hormones. Together they can make you feel 10 to 15 years younger.

So, in addition to lifting your spoon on the Ice Cream Diet, lift some weights, too. Here are two simple, effective exercise routines—one for beginners, the other for more advanced exercisers. *Prevention* recommends that you work up to 20 to 30 minutes of strength training, 2 to 3 days a week, but not on consecutive days. Your muscles need a day's rest in between workouts.

Get yourself a basic set of three pairs of dumbbells in 3, 5, and 8 pounds. For any particular exercise, you should be able to do 8 to 12 repetitions (reps in gym-speak) smoothly, without shaking too much as you finish. And take your time. Each rep should take about 6 seconds. Slowly count "1-2-3" as you lift the weight and again as you lower it.

If you can't do at least 8 reps without shaking, switch to a lighter weight. Once you can easily do more than 12 reps in good form, move up to a heavier weight. Remember, muscles only change when you challenge them.

BEGINNERS WORKOUT: FIRM UP IN THREE EASY MOVES

For this workout, you'll need a pair of dumbbells and an exercise bench or sturdy piece of furniture. Do one set of 8 to 12 reps for each of these exercises, 2 to 3 days a week (but not on consecutive days).

Squat
Stand in front of a chair with your feet about shoulder-width apart. Bending at the knees and hips, slowly lower yourself as though you're sitting. Raise your arms in front of you for better balance. Keep your back straight, and make sure you can always see your toes. Stop just shy of touching the chair. Hold for a second, then stand back up.

Chest Press
Lie on your back on an exercise bench or sturdy piece of furniture, with your knees bent and your feet on the ground. Hold dumbbells just about chest height with your elbows pointing out. Slowly press the dumbbells straight up. Hold for a second, then slowly lower.

Bent-Over Row
Bending at the hips, place your right hand and right knee on a bench or chair. Holding a dumbbell in your left hand, let

that arm hang straight down with your palm facing in. Slowly pull the dumbbell up toward your chest, keeping your elbow and arm close by your side. Hold for a second, then slowly lower. Do one set, then repeat with your right arm.

ADVANCED WORKOUT: BLAST OFF A PLATEAU

You'll need a pair of dumbbells, an exercise band, and a sturdy chair for this routine. Do one set of 10 repetitions of each exercise, resting for 30 to 60 seconds between exercises. Do this workout two to three times a week, allowing a day of rest in between.

Seated Leg Lift

Sit on a sturdy chair with your feet flat on the floor. Slowly lift your lower left leg until it is in line with your thigh. Slowly lower. Do one set, then repeat with your right leg.

Squat

Stand in front of a chair with your feet about shoulder-width apart. Bending at the knees and hips, slowly lower yourself as though you're sitting. Raise your arms in front of you for better balance. Keep your back straight, and make sure you can always see your toes. Stop just shy of touching the chair. Hold for a second, then stand back up.

Hamstring Curl

Lie on your stomach on the floor or a mat with your arms crossed and supporting your head. Flex your feet, so your soles are perpendicular to the floor. Bending your left knee, bring your foot toward your butt until your leg is bent at a 90-degree angle. Keep your hips on the floor and your foot flexed. Slowly lower. Do one set, then repeat with your right leg.

Lunge

Standing with your feet together, step back about 2 to 3 feet with your right foot. Bending your left knee, slowly lower

STRENGTHEN WHILE YOUR ICE CREAM SOFTENS

It's a fact of life. It takes a good 10 minutes for ice cream to soften enough to actually scoop it out into a bowl. Here's a great way to make use of that time. Do these easy, weight-free exercises while waiting in the kitchen for your ice cream to soften.

POWER JUMP

This may be the best exercise for preventing osteoporosis. It builds denser hipbones and more powerful leg muscles.

Simply jump straight up and down for 2 minutes. Don't jump barefoot or with nonathletic shoes, and don't lock your knees when you land. If you feel pain in your back, hips, knees, ankles, or feet, check your position, rest for a few days, or do the move in a shorter range of motion. See your doctor if pain persists.

BICYCLE CRUNCH

It may take some convincing to get you to lie down on your kitchen floor, but the stomach-firming results from this exercise make it worth it! Lie on your back with your legs extended. Place your hands behind your head, but don't interlace your fingers. Tilt your pelvis to press your lower back into the floor. Keeping your elbows out to the sides, slowly bring your head and shoulders off the floor to the count of three by contracting your abdominal muscles. At the same time, bend your right knee and lift your leg toward your chest. Keep your feet relaxed. Hold for 1 second, then slowly lower to the count of three. Repeat with your left leg. Eight to 12 repetitions are considered a set. Do two or three sets, allowing 30 to 60 seconds of rest between sets.

If you feel pain in your lower back or neck, check your position, rest for a few days, or do the move in a shorter range of motion. See your doctor if pain persists.

HEEL RAISE

This exercise tones your lower legs, strengthens calf muscles, and increases the flexibility of your ankle joints. Stand with your feet shoulder-width apart and 1 foot from a wall or counter. Rest your hand(s) lightly on the support to keep your balance. Keep your back straight, head up, and eyes forward. To the count of three, lift your heels off the floor, coming all the way up onto the balls of your feet and your toes. Hold for 1 second. Then to the count of three, slowly lower your heels back to the floor.

If you feel pain in your knee, ankle, heel, or foot, check your position, rest for a few days, or do the move in a shorter range of motion. See your doctor if pain persists.

Use your imagination to adapt other easy, weight-free exercises for the kitchen. Then, enjoy your ice cream!

yourself. Keep your left knee directly over your ankle. Before your right knee touches the floor, push off with your right foot, and return to the starting position. Do one set, then repeat with your left leg.

Pullover

Lie on your back on the floor or a mat. Bend your knees so the soles of your feet are flat on the floor. Grasp dumbbell with both hands and hold it over your chest. Without bending your elbows, lower it backward over your head as far as comfortably possible. Don't arch your back. Slowly return to the starting position.

Lat Pulldown

Sit in a sturdy chair with your feet flat on the floor. Hold an exercise band above your head with your arms straight and your hands about shoulder-width apart. The band should be taut, but not pulled tight. Bending your left arm, pull your elbow down toward your hip. Slowly release. Do one set, then repeat with your right arm.

Chest Fly

Lie on your back on the floor or a mat. Hold dumbbells above your chest with your palms facing each other and your elbows slightly bent. Slowly lower your arms out to the sides and then raise them.

Chest Press

Lie on your back on the floor or a mat. Hold dumbbells just above chest height with your elbows pointing out. Slowly press the dumbbells straight up, extending your arms. Slowly lower.

Biceps Curl

Sit on a sturdy chair with your feet flat on the floor. Holding dumbbells at your sides, palms facing forward, slowly lift the dumbbells toward your chest, then lower.

Seated Row

Sit on the floor with your legs extended straight out in front of you. With your arms extended in front of you, hold an exercise band so it's taut, but not pulled tight. Squeeze your shoulder blades together, and pull your hands back toward your rib cage. Your elbows should be close to your body and pointing back. Slowly release.

Reverse Curl

Lie on your back on the floor or a mat. Bend your hips and knees so that your legs are over your midsection and relaxed. Slowly contract your abdominal muscles, lifting your hips 2 to 4 inches off the floor. Slowly lower.

Diagonal Curl-Up

Lie on your back on the floor or a mat. Interlace your hands behind your head. Bend your knees so your feet are flat on the floor. Slowly lift your head and shoulders off the floor, twist to the left, and bring your right shoulder toward your left knee. Slowly lower. Repeat, alternating sides.

Lateral Raise

Stand with your feet shoulder-width apart. Holding dumbbells at your sides, slowly lift them to almost shoulder height. Keep your elbows slightly bent. Slowly lower.

Overhead Press

Sit on a sturdy chair. Hold dumbbells at shoulder height, elbows bent, palms facing in. Press the dumbbells straight overhead, then slowly lower.

Triceps Kickback

Stand facing a sturdy chair, about a foot away. Rest your right palm on the seat of the chair for balance. Hold a dumbbell with your left arm bent at a 90-degree angle and your elbow at your side. Lifting the dumbbell backward, extend your arm until it is straight. Don't move your upper arm or shoulder. Slowly lower. Do one set, then repeat with your right arm.

AN ICE CREAM COMPARISON

We've created this chart so that you can see at a glance how your favorite ice creams and other frozen desserts stack up in terms of their calorie, total fat, saturated fat, and calcium contents. While the chart contains more than 300 items, it is far from exhaustive. For example, we've included only a selection of products within given brands. And some of the brands are available only in certain parts of the country. We encourage you to check out the regional brands when you do your comparison shopping. And don't forget store brands: Some are excellent!

Remember, for an ice cream or another frozen dessert to fit the Ice Cream Diet guidelines, it should supply 125 calories or less per serving. A calcium content of 100 milligrams (10 percent of the Daily Value) per serving is a plus.

If you choose an ice cream that meets the 125-calorie criteria, the total fat and saturated fat automatically will be low. But you can evaluate the fat content of any ice cream by multiplying the grams of total fat or saturated fat by the number of servings you're planning to have. This will tell you how much fat you'll be getting.

As a rule, women should limit total fat to 50 grams per day, and saturated fat to 11 grams per day. For men, the caps are 66 grams and 15 grams, respectively. So if the ice cream you're considering delivers a major chunk of your daily fat or saturated fat allowance, it should be reserved for an occasional splurge. (For tips on how to splurge without undermining your weight-loss efforts, see chapter 11.)

The nutrition values listed here come from product labels and company Web sites; be aware that they may change. Keep in mind, too, that the values for a given product may vary from one part of the country to another, because of differences in manufacturing processes and restaurant practices. Even seasonal variations can have an effect. That's why you should double-check nutrition values on product labels and company Web sites, just to be sure. The values presented here are for informational purposes only.

BRAND	ITEM	FLAVOR	SERVING SIZE
Baskin Robbins	Hard scooped Premium Ice Cream	Chocolate	Regular scoop (4 fl oz)
		Vanilla	Regular scoop (4 fl oz)
		French Vanilla	Regular scoop (4 fl oz)
		Banana Strawberry	Regular scoop (4 fl oz)
		Chocolate Chip	Regular scoop (4 fl oz)
		Pralines 'n Cream	Regular scoop (4 fl oz)
		Jamoca Almond Fudge	Regular scoop (4 fl oz)
	Hard Scooped Sherbets, Ices, and Sorbets	Rainbow Sherbet	Regular scoop (4 fl oz)
		Daiquiri Ice	Regular scoop (4 fl oz)
		Peachy Keen Sorbet	Regular scoop (4 fl oz)

CALORIES	FAT (GRAMS)	SATURATED FAT (GRAMS)	CALCIUM (PERCENT DV)
270	16	10	6
250	16	10	10
160	10	6	8
130	7	4.5	6
270	17	11	6
280	15	8	6
280	16	8	6
160	2	1.5	4
130	0	0	4
110	0	0	4

BRAND	ITEM	FLAVOR	SERVING SIZE
Baskin Robbins	Hard Scooped Lowfat Ice Cream	Espresso 'n Cream	Regular scoop (4 fl oz)
	Hard Scooped Lowfat Yogurt	Maui Brownie Madness	Regular scoop (4 fl oz)
	Yogurt Gone Crazy	Perils of Praline	Regular scoop (4 fl oz)
		Maui Brownie Madness	Regular scoop (4 fl oz)
		Raspberry Cheese Louise	Regular scoop (4 fl oz)
	Hard Scooped No Sugar Added Ice Cream (Nutrasweet)	Thin Mint	Regular scoop (4 fl oz)
		Peach Crumb Pie	Regular scoop (4 fl oz)
	Soft Serve Nonfat Yogurt	Chocolate	Small
		Chocolate Banana Twist	Small
		Chocolate Mint	Small
		Kahlua	Small
	Soft Serve Truly Free Yogurt (Nutrasweet)	Café Mocha	Small

CALORIES	FAT (GRAMS)	SATURATED FAT (GRAMS)	CALCIUM (PERCENT DV)
180	2.5	1.5	10
250	9	3.5	Not available
140	3	1.5	10
140	3	1	10
130	3	2	10
160	4	3	15
180	5	2.5	10
190	0.5	0	Not available
100	0	0	15
120	0	0	15
110	0	0	15
140	0.5	0.5	Not available

BRAND	ITEM	FLAVOR	SERVING SIZE
Baskin Robbins	Beverages	Chocolate Ice Cream Shake	Regular
		Vanilla Ice Cream Shake	Regular
		Cappuccino Blast (with whipped cream)	Regular
		Very Strawberry Smoothie (with soft serve ice cream)	Regular
Ben and Jerry's	Ice cream	Aloha Macadamia	½ cup
		Apple Crumble	½ cup
		Bovinity Divinity	½ cup
		Cherry Garcia	½ cup
		Chocolate Chip Cookie Dough	½ cup
		Chocolate Fudge Brownie	½ cup
		Chubby Hubby	½ cup
		Chunky Monkey	½ cup
		Coffee Heath Bar Crunch	½ cup
		Concession Obsession	½ cup
		Island Paradise	½ cup
		Kaberry Kaboom	½ cup

CALORIES	FAT (GRAMS)	SATURATED FAT (GRAMS)	CALCIUM (PERCENT DV)
750	43	21	Not available
630	35	22	Not available
340	16	10	Not available
320	1	0.5	Not available
330	21	12	15
280	14	9	10
290	18	13	15
260	16	11	10
300	16	10	10
280	15	10	8
350	21	12	15
310	19	11	8
310	18	12	10
300	18	11	15
240	12	7	10
240	13	9	10

BRAND	ITEM	FLAVOR	SERVING SIZE
Ben and Jerry's		New York Super Fudge Chunk	½ cup
		Nutty Waffle Cone	½ cup
		Peanut Butter Cup	½ cup
		Phish Food	½ cup
		Southern Pecan Pie	½ cup
		Vanilla Heath Bar Crunch	½ cup
		Wavy Gravy	½ cup
		World's Best Chocolate	½ cup
		World's Best Vanilla	½ cup
	2-Twisted Ice Cream	Everything But The . . .	½ cup
		Jerry's Jubilee	½ cup
		Monkey Wrench	½ cup
		S.N.A.F.U.	½ cup
		This is Nuts	½ cup
		Urban Jumble	½ cup
	Yogurt	Cherry Garcia	½ cup
		Chocolate Fudge Brownie	½ cup

CALORIES	FAT (GRAMS)	SATURATED FAT (GRAMS)	CALCIUM (PERCENT DV)
320	21	12	10
310	19	12	15
380	25	13	15
300	14	10	10
290	19	11	15
310	19	10	10
340	20	11	20
280	17	12	15
250	16	10	10
320	19	11	15
260	14	10	15
310	20	10	15
250	14	13	15
300	20	12	15
310	21	11	15
170	3	2	15
190	2.5	1	20

BRAND	ITEM	FLAVOR	SERVING SIZE
Ben and Jerry's		Chocolate Chip Cookie Dough	1/2 cup
		Ooey Gooey Cake	1/2 cup
		Phish Food	1/2 cup
		Raspberry Gone Coconuts	1/2 cup
	Novelties	Cherry Garcia Ice Cream Pop	1 pop
		Cherry Garcia Yogurt Pop	1 pop
		Cookie Dough Pop	1 pop
		Phish Stick	1 stick
		Phish Stick Pop	1 pop
		Vanilla Heath Bar Crunch Pop	1 pop
		Vanilla Pop	1 pop
Breyer's	Ice Cream	Chocolate	1/2 cup
		Natural Vanilla	1/2 cup
	All Natural Calcium Rich Ice Cream	Vanilla	1/2 cup
	Ice Cream Parlor Ice Cream	Mississippi Mud	1/2 cup
		With Oreo	1/2 cup

CALORIES	FAT (GRAMS)	SATURATED FAT (GRAMS)	CALCIUM (PERCENT DV)
200	4.5	2.5	8
190	3.5	2	15
230	5	4	15
210	5	1.5	15
250	16	10	8
250	13	8	20
410	24	11	15
290	18	11	8
260	16	10	8
320	21	13	15
330	22	14	15
160	9	5	6
150	9	5	8
130	7	4	30
180	9	5	6
160	8	4.5	8

BRAND	ITEM	FLAVOR	SERVING SIZE
Breyer's		With Reese's Peanut Butter Cups	½ cup
		Strawberry Shortcake	½ cup
	All Natural Light Ice Cream	Vanilla	½ cup
		Chocolate Strawberry Vanilla	½ cup
		French Vanilla	½ cup
	Fat-Free Ice Creams	Vanilla	½ cup
	No Sugar Added Light Ice Cream	Vanilla	½ cup
		Chocolate Strawberry Vanilla	½ cup
	No Sugar Added Light Ice Cream	Vanilla Fudge Twirl	½ cup
	All Natural Fruit Sherbet	Natural Orange	½ cup
		Rainbow (orange, raspberry, tropical)	½ cup
	All Natural Frozen Yogurt	Chocolate	½ cup
		Natural Vanilla	½ cup

CALORIES	FAT (GRAMS)	SATURATED FAT (GRAMS)	CALCIUM (PERCENT DV)
180	9	4.5	8
160	6	4	8
120	3	2	10
110	3	2	10
120	4	2	15
90	0	0	10
90	4.5	2.5	10
90	4.5	2.5	10
100	4.5	2.5	10
120	1.5	1	4
120	1.5	1	4
150	4.5	3	10
140	4.5	3	10

BRAND	ITEM	FLAVOR	SERVING SIZE
Breyer's		Vanilla, Chocolate, Strawberry	½ cup
	Novelties	Viennetta	1 slice
Burger King	Pie	Hershey's Sundae Pie	1 slice
	Shakes	Chocolate	Small
		Strawberry	Small
		Vanilla	Small
Carvel	Ice Cream	Chocolate	4 fl oz
		Vanilla	4 fl oz
	No Fat Ice Cream	Chocolate	4 fl oz
		Vanilla	4 fl oz
	Sherbet	Various	4 fl oz
	No Sugar Added	Vanilla	4 fl oz
Dairy Queen	Cones	DQ Vanilla Soft Serve	½ cup
		DQ Chocolate Soft Serve	½ cup
		Vanilla cone	Small
		Chocolate cone	Small
		Dipped cone	Small
s	Beverages	Chocolate Malt	Small
		Chocolate Shake	Small

CALORIES	FAT (GRAMS)	SATURATED FAT (GRAMS)	CALCIUM (PERCENT DV)
120	2.5	1.5	10
190	11	7	10
310	18	13	4
340	6	4	25
390	6	4	35
330	6	4	35
190	10	6	15
200	10	6	15
120	0	0	8
120	0	0	15
140	1	0.5	4
130	3	2	15
140	4.5	3	15
150	5	3.5	10
230	7	4.5	20
240	8	5	15
340	17	9	20
650	16	10	45
560	15	10	45

BRAND	ITEM	FLAVOR	SERVING SIZE
Dairy Queen		Frozen Hot Chocolate	1
		Misty Slush	Small
	Sundaes	Chocolate Sundae	Small
	Royal Treats	Banana Split	1
		Peanut Buster Parfait	1
		Pecan Mudslide	1
		Strawberry Shortcake	1
		Brownie Earthquake	1
	Novelties	DQ Sandwich	1
		Chocolate Dilly Bar	1
		Buster Bar	1
		Starkiss	1
		DQ Fudge Bar— No Sugar Added	1
		DQ Vanilla Orange Bar— No Sugar Added	1
		Lemon DQ Freez'r	1/2 cup
	Blizzard Flavor Treats	Chocolate Sandwich Cookie Blizzard	Small

CALORIES	FAT (GRAMS)	SATURATED FAT (GRAMS)	CALCIUM (PERCENT DV)
860	35	16	45
220	0	0	0
280	7	4.5	20
510	12	8	25
730	31	17	30
650	30	12	30
430	14	9	25
740	27	16	25
200	6	3	8
210	13	7	10
450	28	12	15
80	0	0	0
50	0	0	10
60	0	0	6
80	0	0	0
520	18	9	35

BRAND	ITEM	FLAVOR	SERVING SIZE
Dairy Queen		Chocolate Chip Cookie Dough Blizzard	Small
	DQ Treatzza Pizza and Cake	Heath DQ Treatzza Pizza	1/8 of Pizza
		M&Ms DQ Treatzza Pizza	1/8 of Pizza
		DQ Frozen 8" Round Cake (undecorated)	1/8 of cake
		DQ Layered 8" Round Cake (undecorated)	1/8 of cake
Denali	Denali Alaskan Classics Ice Cream	Bear Claw	1/2 cup
		Caramel Caribou	1/2 cup
		Glacier Mint	1/2 cup
		Iditarod Peanut Butter	1/2 cup
		Moosetracks	1/2 cup
		Wolf Pack Cherry	1/2 cup
Dippin' Dots	Ice Cream	Various flavors	5 oz
	Non-Fat Yogurt	Various flavors	5 oz
	No Sugar Added Reduced Fat Ice Cream	Vanilla	5 oz
	Fat-Free/ No Sugar Added	Fudge	5 oz

CALORIES	FAT (GRAMS)	SATURATED FAT (GRAMS)	CALCIUM (PERCENT DV)
660	24	13	35
180	7	3.5	6
190	7	4	6
370	13	6	20
330	12	8	20
170	9	5	8
170	9	6	8
170	9	5	8
170	10	6	8
200	13	6	8
170	10	4.5	8
190	9	6	10
110	0	0	8
120	4	2.5	10
60	0	0	8

BRAND	ITEM	FLAVOR	SERVING SIZE
Dippin' Dots	Flavored Ice	Various flavors	5 oz
	Flavored Sherbet	Various flavors	5 oz
Dole	Fruit Dips Creamy Fruit Bar	Banana	1 bar
Dove	Bars	Milk Chocolate with Vanilla Ice Cream	1 bar
		Original Dove Chocolate with Vanilla Ice Cream	1 bar
Dreyer's Dreamery	Ice Cream	Black Raspberry Avalanche	½ cup
		Caramel Toffee Bar Heaven	½ cup
		Chocolate Peanut Butter Chunk	½ cup
		Chocolate Truffle Explosion	½ cup
		Cool Mint	½ cup
		Deep Dish Apple Pie	½ cup
		Dulce de Leche	½ cup
		Grandma's Cookie Jar	½ cup
		Vanilla	½ cup

CALORIES	FAT (GRAMS)	SATURATED FAT (GRAMS)	CALCIUM (PERCENT DV)
50	0	0	0
100	1	1	4
190	9	6	6
260	17	11	10
260	17	11	6
250	14	9	10
270	14	8	10
310	18	9	10
280	15	9	10
280	14	10	8
280	15	9	8
270	14	9	10
270	14	7	10
260	15	9	15

BRAND	ITEM	FLAVOR	SERVING SIZE
Edy's	Frozen Yogurt	Black Cherry Vanilla Swirl	1/2 cup
		Caramel Praline Crunch	1/2 cup
		Raspberry	1/2 cup
		Vanilla	1/2 cup
	Grand Ice Cream	Butter Pecan	1/2 cup
		Cherry Chocolate Chip	1/2 cup
		French Vanilla	1/2 cup
		Ice Cream Sandwich	1/2 cup
		Mint Chocolate Chips!	1/2 cup
		Neapolitan	1/2 cup
		Vanilla	1/2 cup
		Vanilla Chocolate	1/2 cup
	Grand Light Ice Cream	French Silk	1/2 cup
		Vanilla	1/2 cup
	Home Made Ice Cream	All Natural Vanilla	1/2 cup
		Double Chocolate Chunk	1/2 cup
		Old Fashioned Butter Pecan	1/2 cup

CALORIES	FAT (GRAMS)	SATURATED FAT (GRAMS)	CALCIUM (PERCENT DV)
90	0	0	30
100	0	0	30
90	2.5	1.5	20
90	0	0	30
170	10	5	6
160	8	5	6
160	9	5	6
150	7	4.5	6
170	9	6	6
140	7	4.5	6
140	8	5	6
150	8	4.5	6
130	4.5	3	6
100	3	2	6
130	7	4.5	6
170	9	6	6
160	10	4.5	6

BRAND	ITEM	FLAVOR	SERVING SIZE
Edy's	No Sugar Added Fat-Free Ice Cream	Blueberry Cobbler	½ cup
		Chocolate Fudge	½ cup
		Raspberry Vanilla Swirl	½ cup
		Vanilla	½ cup
	No Sugar Added Light Ice Cream	All About PB	½ cup
		Butter Pecan	½ cup
		Triple Chocolate	½ cup
	No Sugar Added Ice Cream	Chocolate	½ cup
	Whole Fruit Bars	Creamy Banana	1 bar
		Creamy Coconut	1 bar
		Creamy Strawberry	1 bar
		Lemonade	1 bar
		Lime	1 bar
		Strawberry	1 bar
Eskimo Pie	Ice Cream	Vanilla/ Chocolate/ Strawberry	½ cup
	Reduced Fat Ice Cream	Butter Pecan	½ cup
		Fudge Ripple	½ cup

CALORIES	FAT (GRAMS)	SATURATED FAT (GRAMS)	CALCIUM (PERCENT DV)
100	0	0	6
100	0	0	8
90	0	0	8
90	0	0	8
130	6	2	6
110	5	2	6
100	3.5	2	6
100	0	0	8
190	10	7	6
120	3	2.5	8
190	10	7	6
80	0	0	0
80	0	0	0
80	0	0	0
110	4	2.5	15
130	7	3	15
110	4	2.5	15

BRAND	ITEM	FLAVOR	SERVING SIZE
Eskimo Pie		Vanilla	½ cup
	Ice Cream Bars	Dark Chocolate Coated Vanilla	1 bar
		Milk Chocolate Coated Vanilla	1 bar
		Peppermint Patty	1 bar
	No Sugar Added Ice Cream Bars	Milk Chocolate Coated Vanilla	1 bar
	Pudding Bars	Chocolate, vanilla, or chocolate-vanilla swirl	1 bar
	No Sugar Added Reduced Fat Ice Cream Sandwich	Vanilla	1 sandwich
Friendly's	Ice Cream Shoppe Sundaes	Forbidden Chocolate Brownie Sundae	1 container
		Original Fudge Sundae	1 container
		Reese's Pieces Peanut Butter Cup Sundae	1 container
	Candy Shoppe Sundae	Snickers Bar Sundae	1 container
	Red White and Blue Swirls	Vanilla Ice Cream with red raspberry and blue marshmallow swirls	½ cup
	Premium Ice Cream	Butter Crunch	½ cup

CALORIES	FAT (GRAMS)	SATURATED FAT (GRAMS)	CALCIUM (PERCENT DV)
110	4	2.5	15
160	10	8	6
160	11	9	6
250	16	12	8
120	8	6	8
80	1.5	1	10
160	4	2	10
380	18	12	12
310	14	10	10
430	23	12	15
380	17	12	12
160	7	5	6
160	7	5	6

BRAND	ITEM	FLAVOR	SERVING SIZE
Friendly's		Chocolate Chip Cookie Dough	½ cup
		Chocolate 'n Vanilla	½ cup
		Purely Pistachio	½ cup
		Vanilla Chocolate Strawberry	½ cup
	Frozen Yogurt	Fabulous Fudge Swirl	½ cup
		Fudge Berry Swirl	½ cup
	Nonfat Frozen Yogurt	Simply Vanilla	½ cup
Godiva	Ice Cream	Belgian Dark Chocolate	4 oz
		Chocolate Cheesecake	4 oz
		Chocolate with Chocolate Hearts	4 oz
		Chocolate Raspberry Truffle	4 oz
		Classic Milk Chocolate	4 oz
		Vanilla Caramel Pecan	4 oz
		Vanilla with Chocolate Caramel Hearts	4 oz
		White Chocolate Raspberry	4 oz

CALORIES	FAT (GRAMS)	SATURATED FAT (GRAMS)	CALCIUM (PERCENT DV)
170	8	5	6
150	8	5	8
160	9	5	8
140	8	5	8
140	4	2.5	15
150	4	3	10
110	0	0	15
280	17	10	8
310	17	10	10
330	20	13	10
290	16	9	8
290	18	11	10
290	16	9	10
310	18	11	10
260	12	7	10

BRAND	ITEM	FLAVOR	SERVING SIZE
Good Humor	Ice Cream Bars	Cookies & Cream	1 bar
		Chocolate Éclair	1 bar
	Fudgiscle Bars	Fat-Free Fudgsicle Bar	1 bar
		No Sugar Added Fudgsicle Bar	1 bar
		Original Fudgsicle Bar	1 bar
Green's	Premium Ice Cream	Chocolate	1/2 cup
		French Vanilla	1/2 cup
		Peanut Butter Twirl	1/2 cup
		Strawberry	1/2 cup
		Vanilla	1/2 cup
	Lowfat Frozen Yogurt	Mocha Chocolate Chip	1/2 cup
		Vanilla	1/2 cup
	Nonfat Frozen Yogurt	Chocolate Flavored	1/2 cup
		Strawberry	1/2 cup
Häagen-Dazs	Ice cream	Butter Pecan	1/2 cup
		Chocolate	1/2 cup
		Chocolate Peanut Butter	1/2 cup
		Cherry Vanilla	1/2 cup

CALORIES	FAT (GRAMS)	SATURATED FAT (GRAMS)	CALCIUM (PERCENT DV)
190	12	6	6
160	8	3	4
60	0	0	10
45	1	0.5	8
60	1	0.5	6
140	8	4.5	8
150	8	5	8
180	11	5	8
140	7	4.5	8
150	8	5	10
120	3.5	2	10
120	2.5	1.5	10
100	0	0	15
110	0	0	10
310	23	11	10
270	18	11	15
360	24	11	10
240	15	9	10

BRAND	ITEM	FLAVOR	SERVING SIZE
Häagen-Dazs		Coffee	½ cup
		Cookie Dough Chip	½ cup
		Dulce de Leche	½ cup
		Macadamia Brittle	½ cup
		Pineapple Coconut	½ cup
		Rum Raisin	½ cup
		Strawberry	½ cup
		Vanilla	½ cup
		Vanilla Fudge	½ cup
		Vanilla Swiss Almond	½ cup
	Gelato	Chocolate	½ cup
		Raspberry	½ cup
		Tiramisu	½ cup
	Frozen Yogurt	Chocolate Chocolate Chip	½ cup
		Coffee	½ cup
		Vanilla	½ cup
		Vanilla Raspberry Swirl	½ cup
	Nonfat Frozen Yogurt	Strawberry	½ cup
	Sorbet	Chocolate	½ cup

CALORIES	FAT (GRAMS)	SATURATED FAT (GRAMS)	CALCIUM (PERCENT DV)
270	18	11	15
310	20	12	10
290	17	10	15
300	20	12	15
230	13	8	10
270	17	10	10
250	16	10	15
270	18	11	15
290	18	12	15
300	20	11	10
240	8	4.5	15
240	7	3.5	15
250	10	6	15
230	7	4	20
200	4.5	2.5	20
200	4.5	2.5	25
170	2.5	1.5	10
140	0	0	15
120	0	0	0

BRAND	ITEM	FLAVOR	SERVING SIZE
Häagen-Dazs		Orange	½ cup
		Orchard Peach	½ cup
		Raspberry	½ cup
		Strawberry	½ cup
		Zesty Lemon	½ cup
	Ice Cream Bars	Raspberry Sorbet and Vanilla Frozen Yogurt	1 bar
		Chocolate and Dark Chocolate Ice Cream Bars	1 bar
		Dulce de Leche Ice Cream Bars	1 bar
		Vanilla & Almonds Ice Cream Bars	1 bar
		Vanilla & Milk Chocolate Ice Cream Bars	1 bar
	Nonfat Frozen Yogurt Bars	Fat Free Raspberry Vanilla	1 bar
Healthy Choice	Premium Low-fat Ice Cream	Mint Chocolate Chip	½ cup
		Peanut Butter Cup	½ cup
		Rocky Road	½ cup
		Tin Roof Sundae	½ cup
		Vanilla	½ cup

CALORIES	FAT (GRAMS)	SATURATED FAT (GRAMS)	CALCIUM (PERCENT DV)
120	0	0	0
130	0	0	0
120	0	0	0
120	0	0	0
120	0	0	0
90	0	0	6
350	24	25	10
300	19	12	10
380	28	14	10
340	24	14	15
90	0	0	6
120	2	1	10
110	2	1	10
130	2	1	10
120	2	1	10
100	2	1	6

BRAND	ITEM	FLAVOR	SERVING SIZE
Healthy Choice		Cappuccino Chocolate Chunk	½ cup
		Cherry Chocolate Chunk	½ cup
	Low-Fat No Sugar Added Ice Creams	Chocolate Fudge Brownie	½ cup
		Mint Chocolate Chip	½ cup
		Coffee Almond Fudge	½ cup
Kemp	Party Slices	Vanilla	1 slice
Kentucky Fried Chicken	Little Bucket Parfaits	Fudge Brownie	1 parfait
		Lemon Creme	1 parfait
		Chocolate Creme	1 parfait
		Strawberry Shortcake	1 parfait
Klondike	Ice Cream Cones	Big Bear	1 cone
	Ice Cream Bars	Heath Bar	1 bar
		Krunch	1 bar
		Neapolitan	1 bar
		Oreo	1 bar
		York Peppermint Pattie	1 bar
		No Sugar Added Reduced Fat Vanilla	1 bar

CALORIES	FAT (GRAMS)	SATURATED FAT (GRAMS)	CALCIUM (PERCENT DV)
120	2	1	10
110	2	1	10
110	2	1	10
100	2	1	10
110	2	1	10
130	7	4	12
280	10	3.5	2
410	14	8	20
290	15	11	4
200	7	6	2
350	21	8	10
300	20	14	10
290	19	13	10
280	19	14	10
240	10	4	6
290	20	13	10
190	10	7	15

BRAND	ITEM	FLAVOR	SERVING SIZE
Lactaid	Premium Ice Creams	Classic Vanilla	½ cup
		Double Chocolate Chip	½ cup
M&M Mars	Novelties	Snickers Ice Cream Bars	1 bar
		M&M Ice Cream Sandwich	1 sandwich
McDonald's	Parfaits	Fruit 'n Yogurt (with granola)	1 parfait
		Fruit 'n Yogurt Parfait (without granola)	1 parfait
	Cone	Vanilla Reduced Fat	1 cone
	Sundaes	Strawberry	1 sundae
		Hot Caramel	1 sundae
		Hot Fudge	1 sundae
	McFlurry	Butterfinger	1 McFlurry
		M&M	1 McFlurry
		Nestlé Crunch	1 McFlurry
		Oreo	1 McFlurry
	Shakes	Vanilla	Small
		Chocolate	Small
		Strawberry	Small

CALORIES	FAT (GRAMS)	SATURATED FAT (GRAMS)	CALCIUM (PERCENT DV)
160	9	6	8
180	10	6	8
180	11	6	6
250	12	5	4
380	5	2	30
280	4	2	25
150	4.5	3	10
290	7	5	20
360	10	6	25
340	12	9	25
620	22	14	45
630	23	15	50
630	24	16	50
570	20	12	45
360	9	6	35
360	9	6	35
360	9	6	35

BRAND	ITEM	FLAVOR	SERVING SIZE
Mister Cookie Face	Ice Cream Sandwiches	Chocolate and Vanilla Swirl	1 sandwich
		Vanilla	1 sandwich
Nestlé	Bon Bons Premium Bite Size Ice Cream Treats		8 pieces
	Carnation Ice Cream Sandwiches	Vanilla	1
	Drumstick, Sundae Cone	Vanilla	1 cone
	Crunch Ice Cream Bars	Reduced Fat, Vanilla	1 bar
		Vanilla	1 bar
	Nesquick Icescreamers Pops	Milk chocolate & vanilla	1 pop
Popsicle	Ice Cream Bars	Sprinklers	1 bar
Rita's Italian Ice	Ice Cream Cone	Various flavors	Small
	Gelati	Various flavors	Small
	Regular Misto	Various flavors	Regular
	Small Custard	Various flavors	Small
Silhouette "The Skinny Cow"	Fat-Free Fudge Bars	Fudge	1 bar
	Lowfat Ice Cream Sandwich 98% fat-free	Chocolate	1 sandwich

CALORIES	FAT (GRAMS)	SATURATED FAT (GRAMS)	CALCIUM (PERCENT DV)
240	10	6	10
250	11	7	10
330	21	15	8
200	7	3	4
350	19	10	8
140	8	6	4
220	14	10	6
100	4	3	10
130	6	2.5	4
204	3	Not Available	Not Available
380	12	Not Available	Not Available
415	7	Not Available	Not Available
274	15	Not Available	Not Available
60	0	0	0
130	2	1	8

BRAND	ITEM	FLAVOR	SERVING SIZE
Silhouette "The Skinny Cow"	Lowfat Ice Cream Sandwich 98% fat-free	Vanilla	1 sandwich
Starbucks	Frappuccino Coffee Bars	Mocha	1 bar
	Ice Cream	Classic Coffee	½ cup
		Coffee Almond Fudge	½ cup
		Java Chip	½ cup
		Low Fat Latte	½ cup
Taco Bell	Novelty	Chocolate Taco	1
TCBY	Soft Serve Nonfat Frozen Yogurt	Top 6 soft serve nonfat frozen yogurt flavors: Golden Vanilla, White Chocolate Mousse, Dutch Chocolate, Old Fashion Vanilla, Chocolate, Strawberries and Cream	½ cup
	Soft Serve No Sugar Added Nonfat Frozen Yogurt (contains phenylalanine)	Top 4 no sugar added/nonfat flavors: Vanilla, Chocolate, White Chocolate Macadamia Nut, Strawberry	½ cup
	Soft Serve 96% Fat-Free Frozen Yogurt	Various	½ cup

CALORIES	FAT (GRAMS)	SATURATED FAT (GRAMS)	CALCIUM (PERCENT DV)
130	2	1	8
120	2	1	10
230	12	7	10
250	13	7	10
250	13	8	10
170	3	1.5	10
290	16	8	6
110	0	0	10
80	0	0	10
130	3	2	8

BRAND	ITEM	FLAVOR	SERVING SIZE
TCBY	Soft Serve Sorbet	Various	½ cup
	Hand-Dipped Lowfat Ice Cream	Top 4 lowfat ice cream flavors: Raspberry Cheesecake, Banana Pudding, Mint Chocolate Chip, Peanut Butter Fudge Nut	½ cup
	Hand-Dipped No Sugar Added Lowfat Ice Cream (contains phenylalanine)	Vanilla	½ cup
	Swirl Bar	Orange	1 bar
	Swirl Bar	Raspberry	1 bar
Tofutti	Non-dairy frozen dessert	Vanilla	½ cup
		Chocolate Supreme	½ cup
		Butter Pecan	½ cup
Tropicana	Ice Cream Bars	Chocolate Dipped Orange 'n Cream Bar	1 bar
		Orange Cream Bar	1 bar
	Orange Juice Bar	Orange Juice	1 bar
Turkey Hill	Premium Ice Cream	Chocolate Peanut Butter Cup	½ cup
		Original Vanilla	½ cup

CALORIES	FAT (GRAMS)	SATURATED FAT (GRAMS)	CALCIUM (PERCENT DV)
100	0	0	0
120	2.5	1.5	10
100	2.5	1.5	10
80	0.5	0.5	20
80	0.5	0.5	20
190	11	2	0
180	11	2	0
220	13	2	0
120	5	2.5	10
70	1	0.5	10
60	0	0	15
180	11	5	8
140	8	5	8

BRAND	ITEM	FLAVOR	SERVING SIZE
Turkey Hill		Rocky Road	½ cup
		Tin Roof Sundae	½ cup
	Light Ice Cream	Vanilla Bean	½ cup
	Frozen Yogurt	Vanilla Bean	½ cup
	Frozen Yogurt	Tin Roof Sundae	½ cup
Weight Watchers	Smart Ones Bars	Chocolate Mousse	1 bar
		Chocolate Treat	1 bar
		Mocha Java	1 bar
		Orange Vanilla Treat	1 bar
	Smart Ones Sandwiches	Vanilla Sandwich	1 sandwich
Welch's	Fruit juice bars	Strawberry, grape, or raspberry	1 bar
Wendy's	Shakes	Frosty	Junior
			Small
			Medium

CALORIES	FAT (GRAMS)	SATURATED FAT (GRAMS)	CALCIUM (PERCENT DV)
170	8	4	8
160	9	5	8
110	3	2	10
110	2.5	1.5	10
140	4.5	2.5	10
40	1	0.5	8
100	0.5	0	8
80	1.5	1	10
40	0.5	0	6
150	3	1	15
45	0	0	0
170	4	2.5	16
330	8	5	31
440	11	7	41

**Eat Peanut Butter Every Day and Lose
All the Weight You Want!**

The Peanut Butter Diet

Holly McCord, M.A., R.D.
Nutrition Editor, *Prevention* Magazine

Recipe Coordinator, Regina Ragone, M.S., R.D.
Food Editor, *Prevention* Magazine

You *can* eat peanut butter every day and still lose weight!
Many health-conscious dieters have shied away from this
tempting treat, but new studies show that peanut butter
can actually lower your risk for heart disease and diabetes and help you shed unwanted pounds. And because
THE PEANUT BUTTER DIET is so satisfying, those
who follow it are more successful at slimming down than
those who choose a traditional low-fat diet.

Dig in and discover:

- *50 fast-and-fabulous recipes*
- *4 weeks of delicious, super-easy meal plans*
- *A day-by-day diet you can stick to—even
  when you're eating out*
- *Fitness strategies to boost your metabolism
  and decrease body fat*
- *Special tips and treats for the whole family*

AVAILABLE WHEREVER BOOKS ARE SOLD FROM
ST. MARTIN'S PAPERBACKS